MEMORY NOTEBOOK OF NURSING

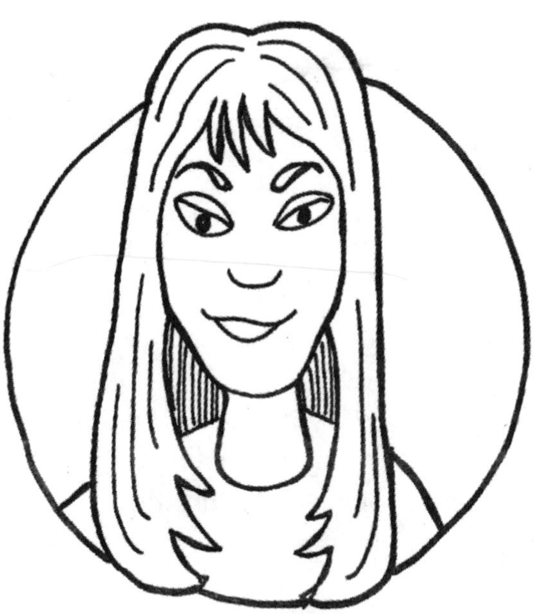

JoAnn Zerwekh, MSN, EdD, RN
Executive Director
Nursing Education Consultants
Ingram, Texas
Nursing Faculty
University of Phoenix
Phoenix, Arizona

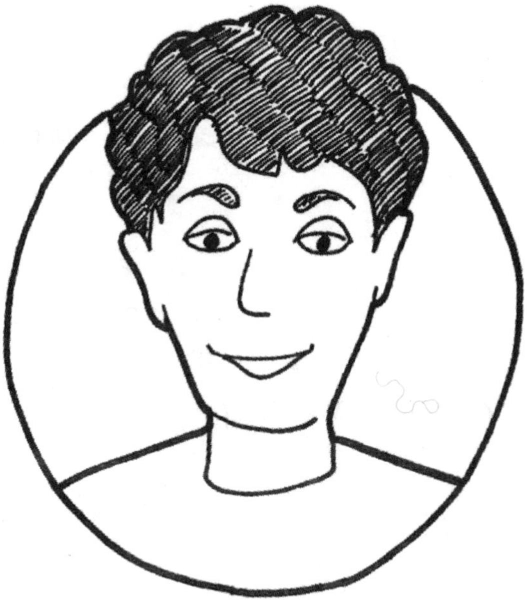

Jo Claborn, MS, RN
Executive Director
Nursing Education Consultants
Ingram, Texas

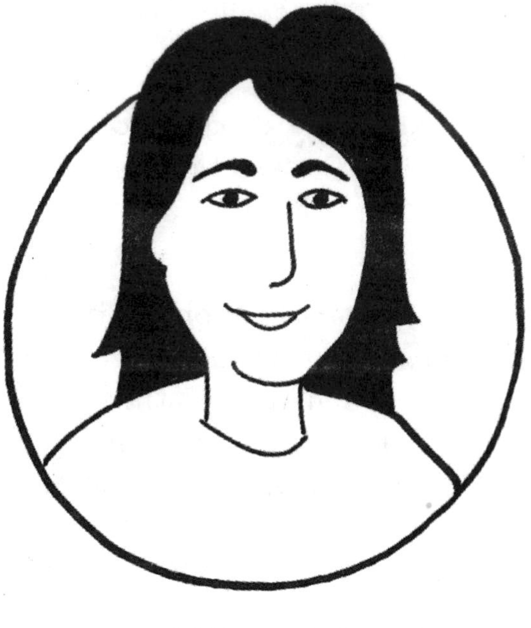

CJ Miller, BSN, RN
Nurse Illustrator
Nursing Education Consultants
Ingram, Texas
Staff Nurse
University of Iowa Hospitals and Clinics
Iowa City, Iowa

Artist: C.J. Miller, RN
Washington, Iowa

Production Manager: Mike Cull
Gingerbread Press, Waxahachie, Texas
Desktop Publishing Assistant: James Halfast
San Angelo, Texas

✦

✦

Printed in the United States of America

Nursing Education Consultants
P O Box 465
Ingram, Texas 78025
(800) 933-7277

ISBN: 1892155133 9781892155139
Library of Congress Catalog Number: 2009925140

✦

Last Digit is the Print Number: 4 3 2 1

Preface

The *Memory Notebook of Nursing: Pharmacology & Diagnostics* has been developed to help you with studying and remembering medications. Thank you for your enthusiastic responses and comments to the 1st edition and we do hope you enjoy this 2nd edition. As before, we have continued to use our style of images that promotes accelerated learning. We are pleased to bring this new edition to you and hope that it helps you to learn new concepts, expand your knowledge base and at times just laugh out loud for the fun of it. We continue to promote the idea that if you can laugh at something, you will remember it. We found ourselves laughing during the revisions.

If you really like this book, then check out *Memory Notebook of Nursing, Vol 1,* and *Memory Notebook of Nursing, Vol 2.* These were the original books in the series, same great concepts, but images and mnemonics for nursing care. Check the inside of the back cover for more information on how and where you can get your copy of each of the *Memory Notebooks of Nursing.*

To assist you in the utilization of this book, here is a little information about accelerated learning and how you can enhance your learning by utilizing both the left (analytical, linear, logical, memory) side of your brain and the right (visual, images, musical, imaginative) side of your brain. Several techniques are used to encourage the whole-brain to think and learn concepts. These techniques are memory tools and mnemonics. Memory tools are aids to assist you to draw associations from other ideas and the use of visual images to help cement the learning. Mnemonics are most often words, phrases, or sentences that help you remember information. As you read over each illustration, get involved with the process and write down your own ideas on the drawings. Think about this – color activates the brain and music increases right brain activity. Involve both sides of your brain when you study. As you are coloring or writing, turn on some music (no words or singing, just instrumental music), don't be afraid to experiment and find out what type of music works for you! You might be very pleasantly surprised with how these activities can promote your retention of information.

We hope you enjoy this 2nd edition of our *Memory Notebook of Nursing: Pharmacology & Diagnostics.* Here is to your continued success on your journey in nursing.

Jo Ann Zerwekh

Jo Carol Claborn

Acknowledgments

We want to acknowledge and thank you the students and faculty for encouraging us to continue with a second edition of the *Memory Notebook of Nursing: Pharmacology & Diagnostics*. Your support and encouragement continue to be the spark that drives us in the production of the *Memory Notebooks*. Your suggestions and ideas continue to make us think and develop more creative images.

We thank our children – Ashley Garneau, Tyler Zerwekh, Jaelyn Conway, Michael Brown and Kimberley Aultman, you continue to give us love and support as we write, rewrite, revise one more book!

JoAnn wishes to thank John Masog for his warm presence in her life, sense of humor and willingness to be a part of it all.

Jo Carol wishes to thank Robert for his continued patience and support of all our activities.

CJ Miller (illustrator) wishes to thank her children Nathan and Kimberley for all their support and encouragement as well as the many great friends that have stayed in her life throughout the years.

Our sincere appreciation to:

James Halfast, our graphics production manager who for many years has juggled NEC with his family and work schedule;

Mike Cull and all the support staff at Gingerbread Press for their patience and support;

Elaine Nokes who keeps our office running smoothly while we are buried in revisions of our books;

Dave Meier from the Center for Accelerated Learning at Lake Geneva, Wisconsin for introducing us to the ideas of accelerated learning;

And to Lucy Claborn – who will be 100 years old this year and continues to inspire us with her humor, courage, and spirit. We love you very much.

Table of Contents

Aminoglycosides

Bad bugs, bad bugs, what ya gonna do??...
What ya gonna do when these
two come for you!!

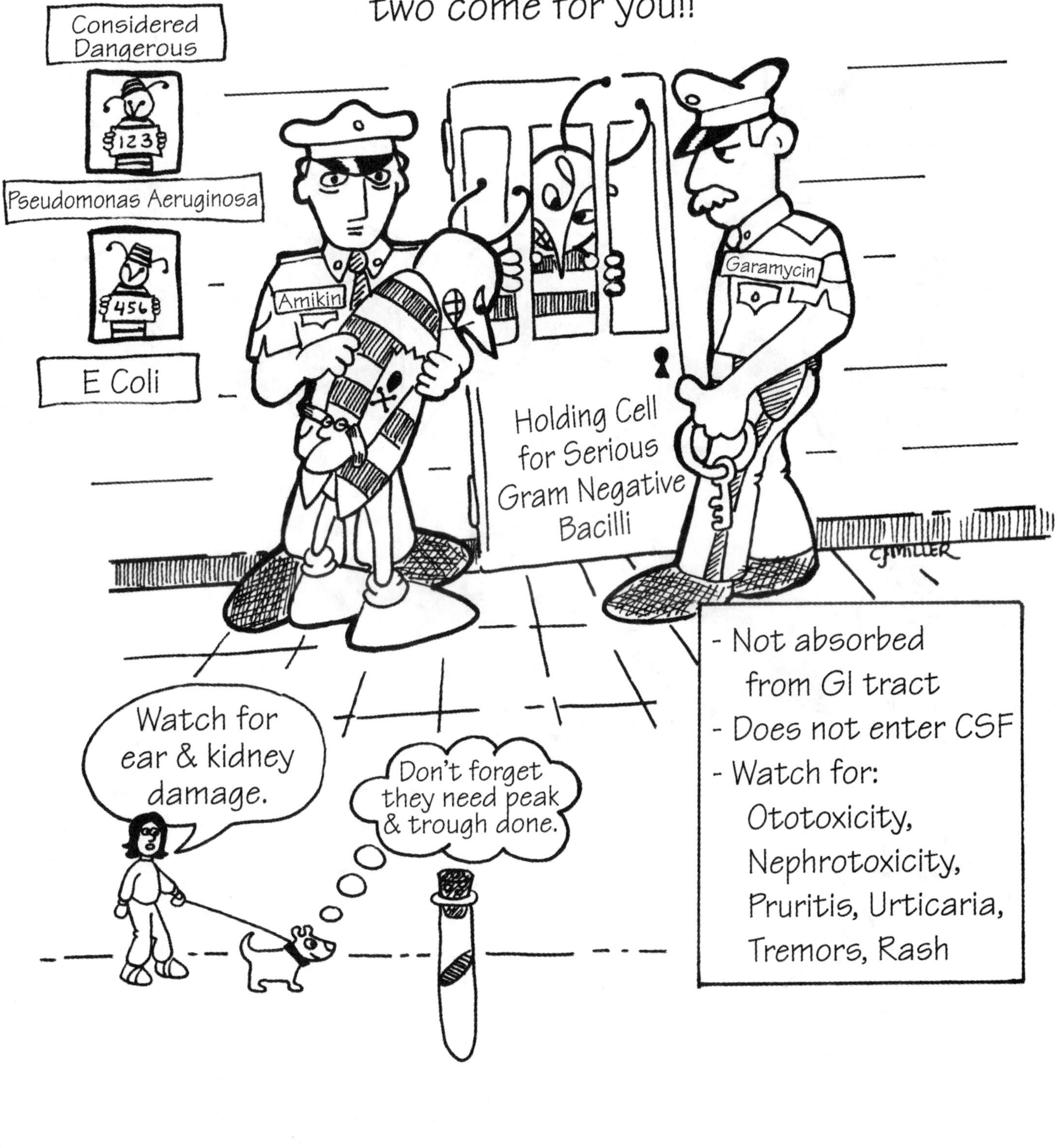

Considered Dangerous
123
Pseudomonas Aeruginosa
456
E Coli
Amikin
Garamycin
Holding Cell for Serious Gram Negative Bacilli
GMILLER
Watch for ear & kidney damage.
Don't forget they need peak & trough done.
- Not absorbed from GI tract
- Does not enter CSF
- Watch for: Ototoxicity, Nephrotoxicity, Pruritis, Urticaria, Tremors, Rash

Amoxicillin

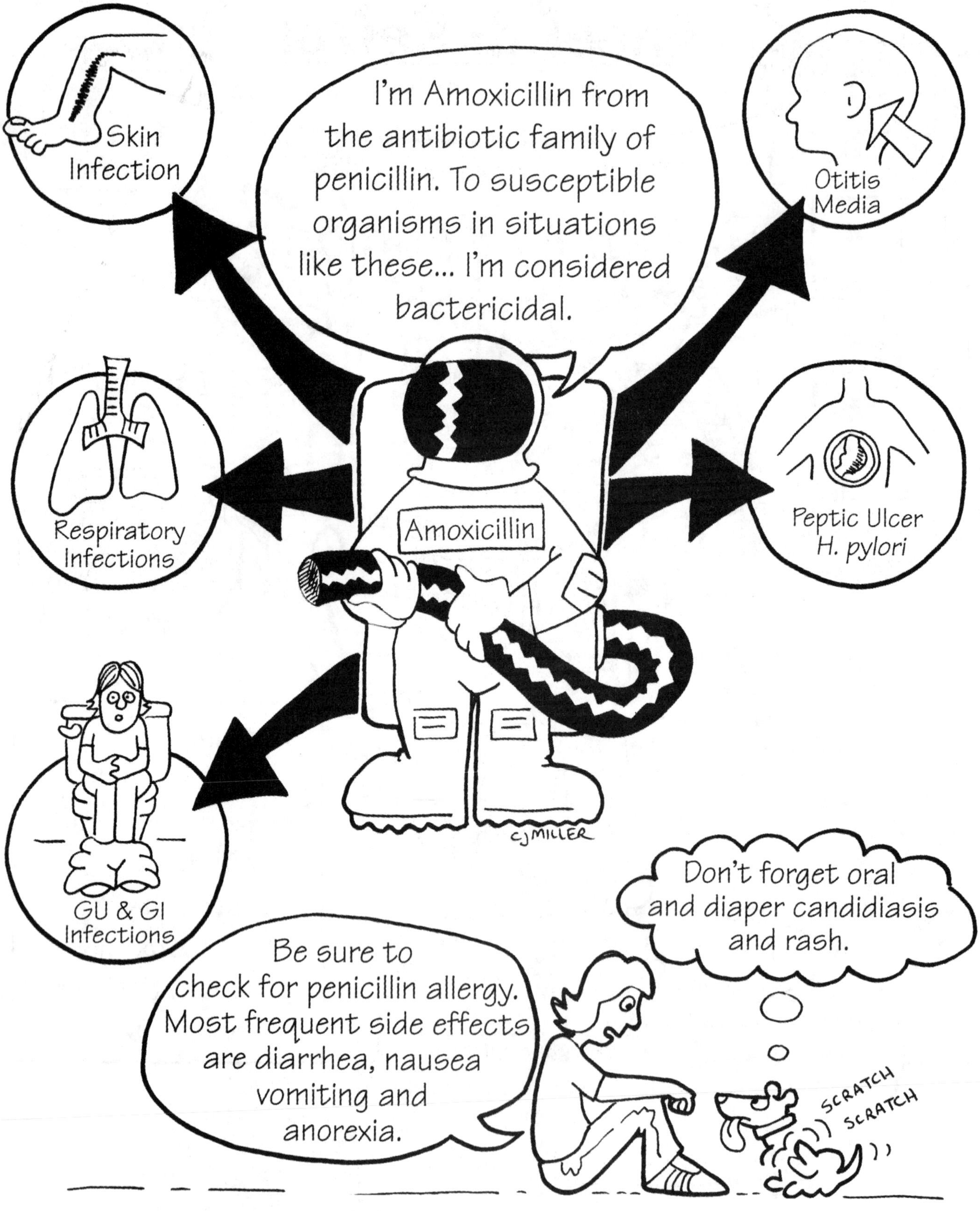
I'm Amoxicillin from the antibiotic family of penicillin. To susceptible organisms in situations like these... I'm considered bactericidal.
Skin Infection
Otitis Media
Respiratory Infections
Amoxicillin
Peptic Ulcer H. pylori
GU & GI Infections
CJMILLER
Don't forget oral and diaper candidiasis and rash.
Be sure to check for penicillin allergy. Most frequent side effects are diarrhea, nausea vomiting and anorexia.
SCRATCH SCRATCH

Ancef & Kefzol

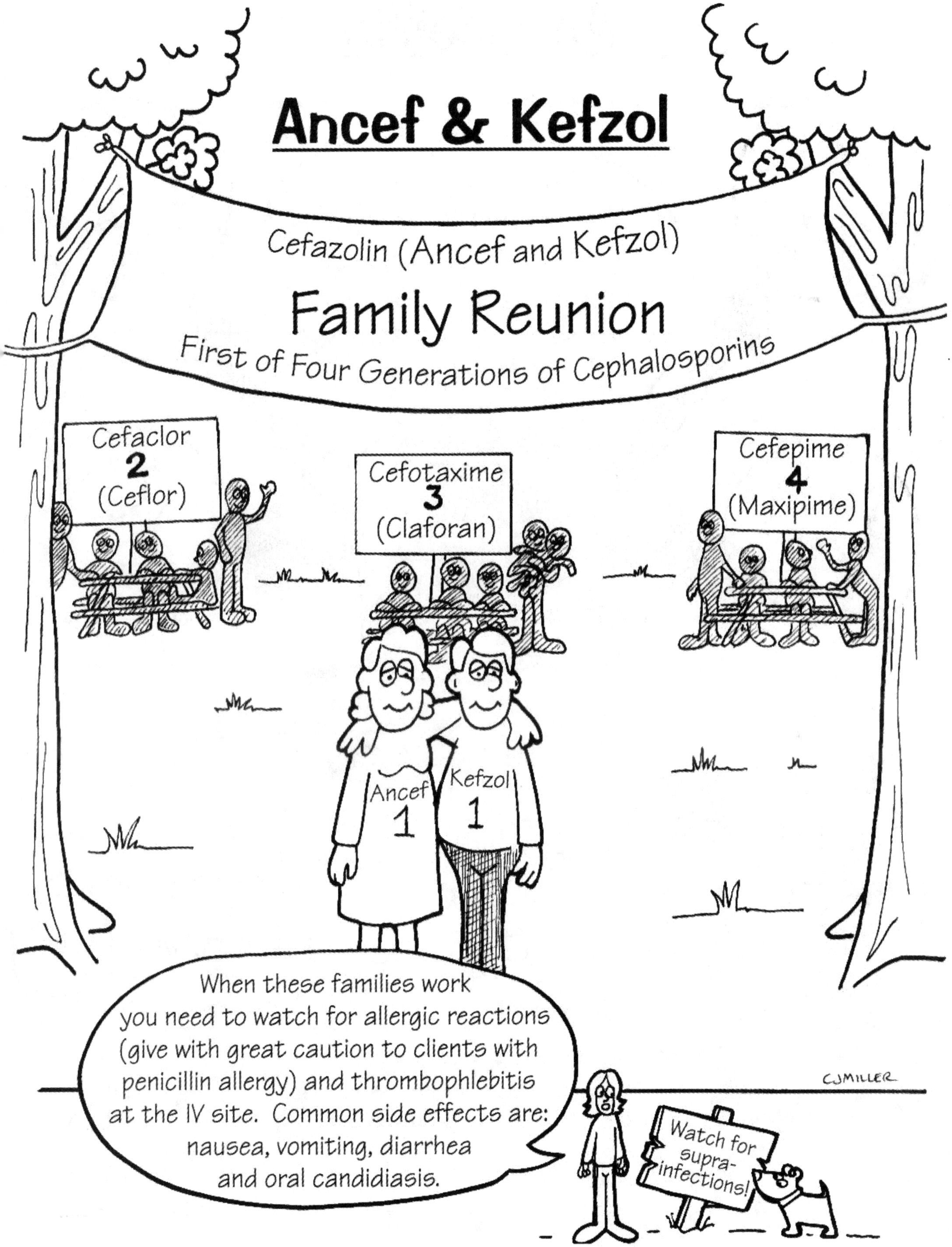
Cefazolin (Ancef and Kefzol)
Family Reunion
First of Four Generations of Cephalosporins
Cefaclor 2 (Ceflor)
Cefotaxime 3 (Claforan)
Cefepime 4 (Maxipime)
Ancef 1
Kefzol 1
When these families work you need to watch for allergic reactions (give with great caution to clients with penicillin allergy) and thrombophlebitis at the IV site. Common side effects are: nausea, vomiting, diarrhea and oral candidiasis.
CJMILLER
Watch for supra-infections!

Antiretrovirals

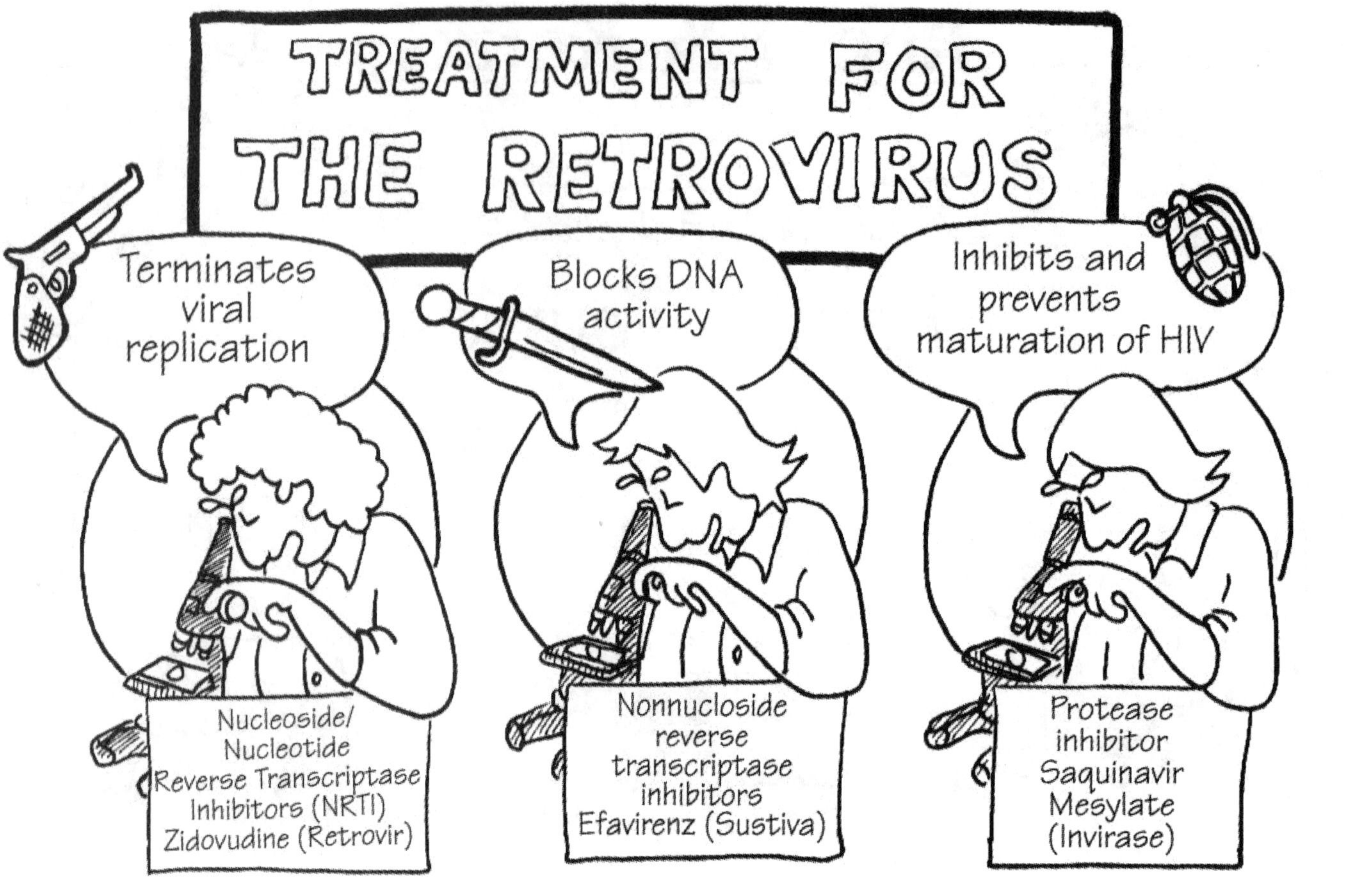
TREATMENT FOR THE RETROVIRUS
Terminates viral replication
Blocks DNA activity
Inhibits and prevents maturation of HIV
Nucleoside/ Nucleotide Reverse Transcriptase Inhibitors (NRTI) Zidovudine (Retrovir)
Nonnucloside reverse transcriptase inhibitors Efavirenz (Sustiva)
Protease inhibitor Saquinavir Mesylate (Invirase)

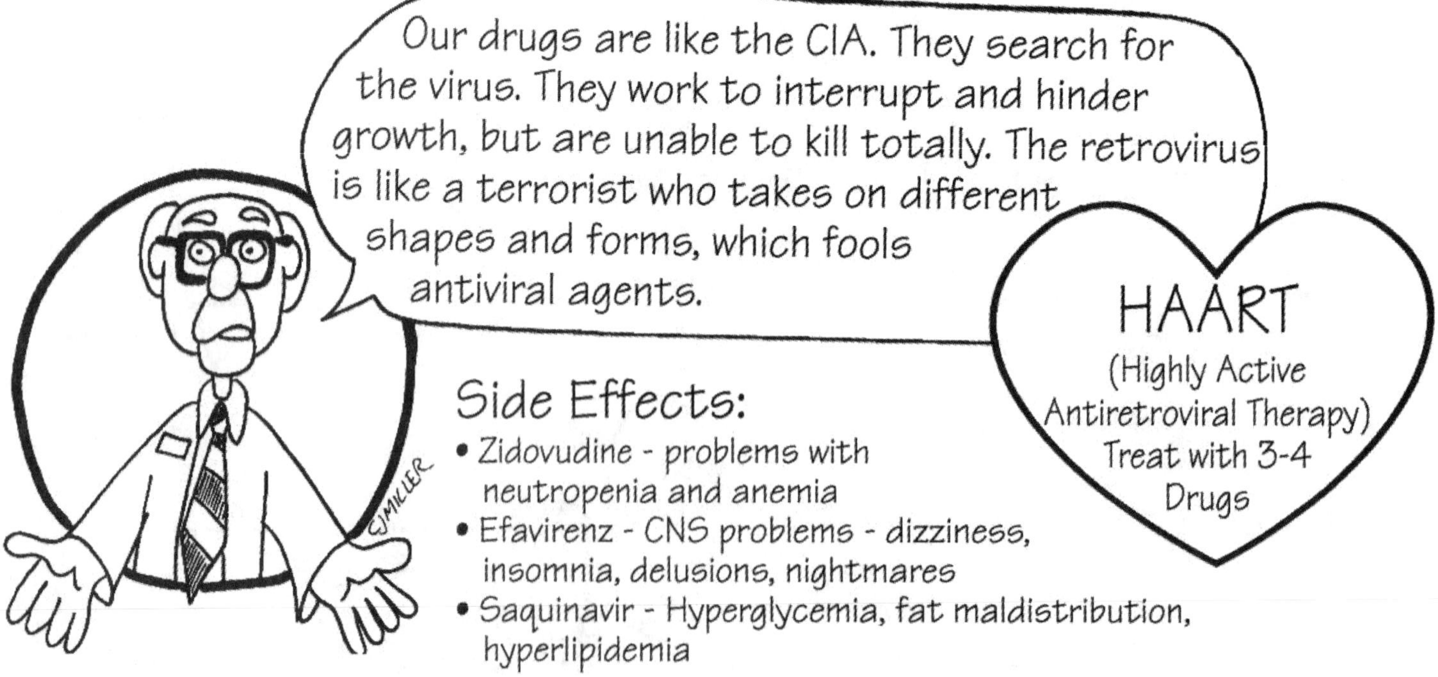
Our drugs are like the CIA. They search for the virus. They work to interrupt and hinder growth, but are unable to kill totally. The retrovirus is like a terrorist who takes on different shapes and forms, which fools antiviral agents.
HAART (Highly Active Antiretroviral Therapy) Treat with 3-4 Drugs
CJMILLER

Side Effects:

- Zidovudine - problems with neutropenia and anemia
- Efavirenz - CNS problems - dizziness, insomnia, delusions, nightmares
- Saquinavir - Hyperglycemia, fat maldistribution, hyperlipidemia

Azithromycin (Zithromax)

Top to Bottom... Mild to Moderate

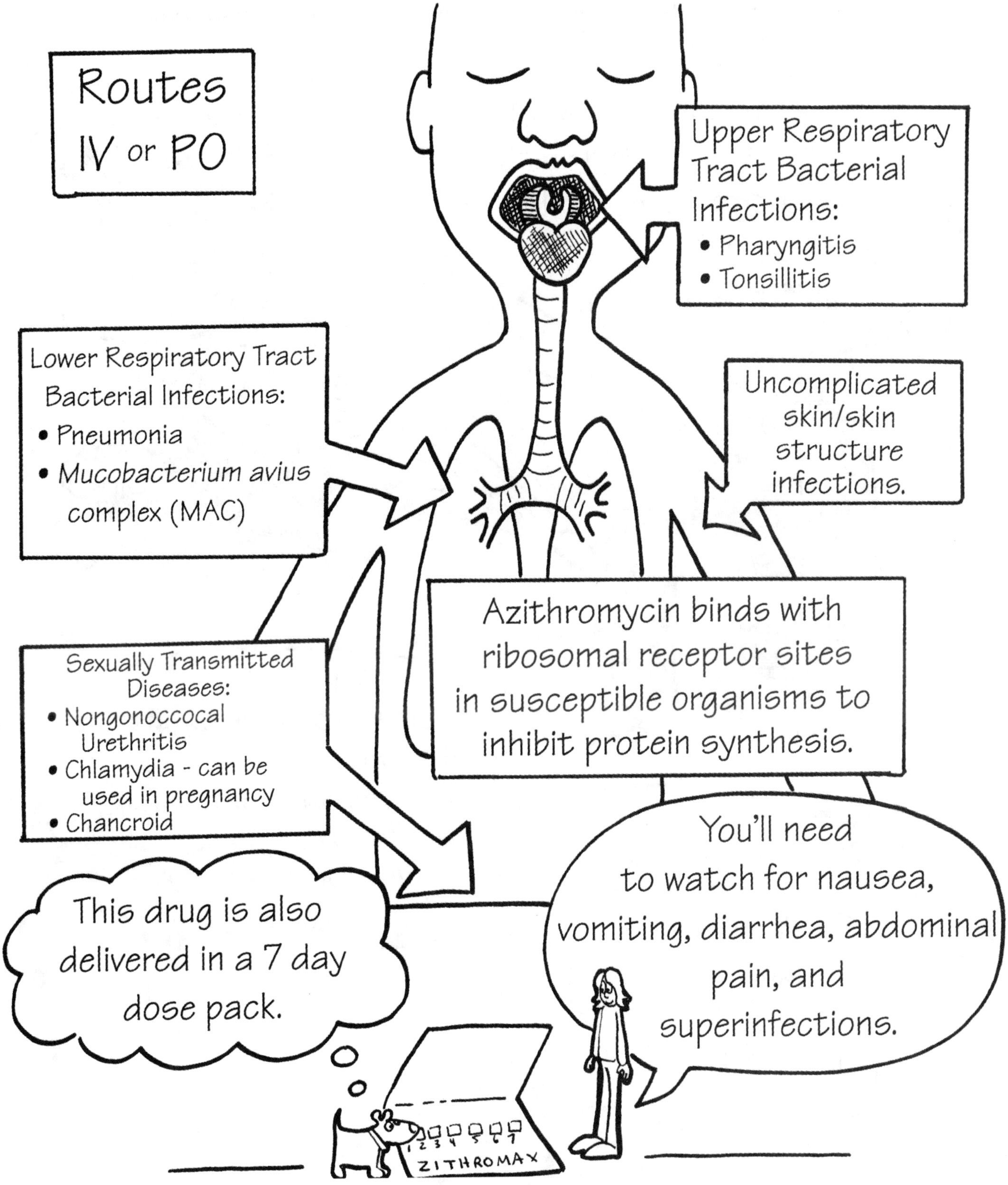

Routes
IV or PO
Upper Respiratory Tract Bacterial Infections:
• Pharyngitis
• Tonsillitis
Lower Respiratory Tract Bacterial Infections:
• Pneumonia
• *Mucobacterium avius* complex (MAC)
Uncomplicated skin/skin structure infections.
Sexually Transmitted Diseases:
• Nongonoccocal Urethritis
• Chlamydia - can be used in pregnancy
• Chancroid
Azithromycin binds with ribosomal receptor sites in susceptible organisms to inhibit protein synthesis.
This drug is also delivered in a 7 day dose pack.
You'll need to watch for nausea, vomiting, diarrhea, abdominal pain, and superinfections.
1 2 3 4 5 6 7
ZITHROMAX

The Azoles

"One Way to Say No to Yeast!"

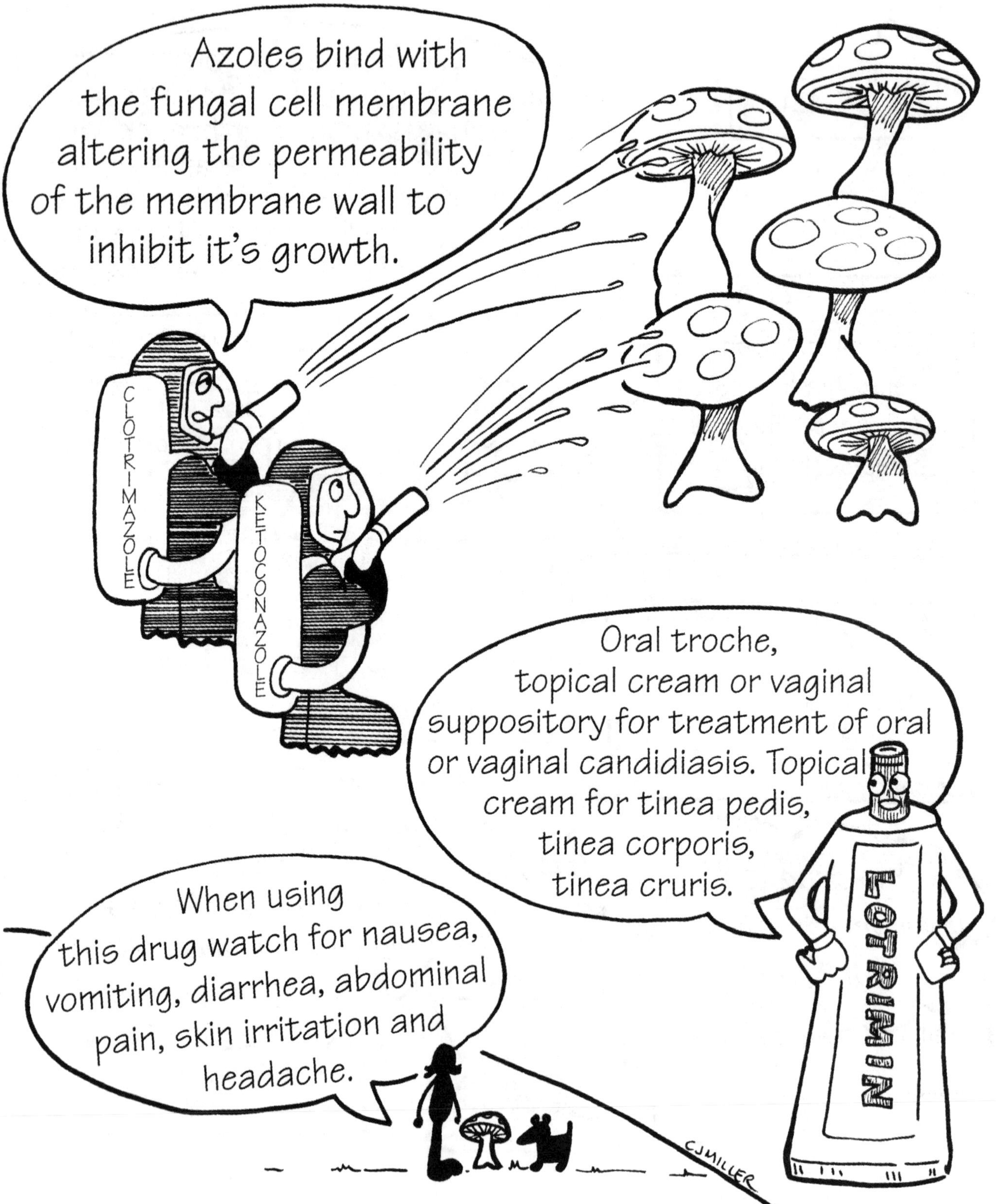
Azoles bind with the fungal cell membrane altering the permeability of the membrane wall to inhibit it's growth.
CLOTRIMAZOLE
KETOCONAZOLE
Oral troche, topical cream or vaginal suppository for treatment of oral or vaginal candidiasis. Topical cream for tinea pedis, tinea corporis, tinea cruris.
LOTRIMIN
When using this drug watch for nausea, vomiting, diarrhea, abdominal pain, skin irritation and headache.
CJMILLER

Rocephin

"A heavy duty 3rd Generation Cephalosporin - does the job against bacterial infections!"

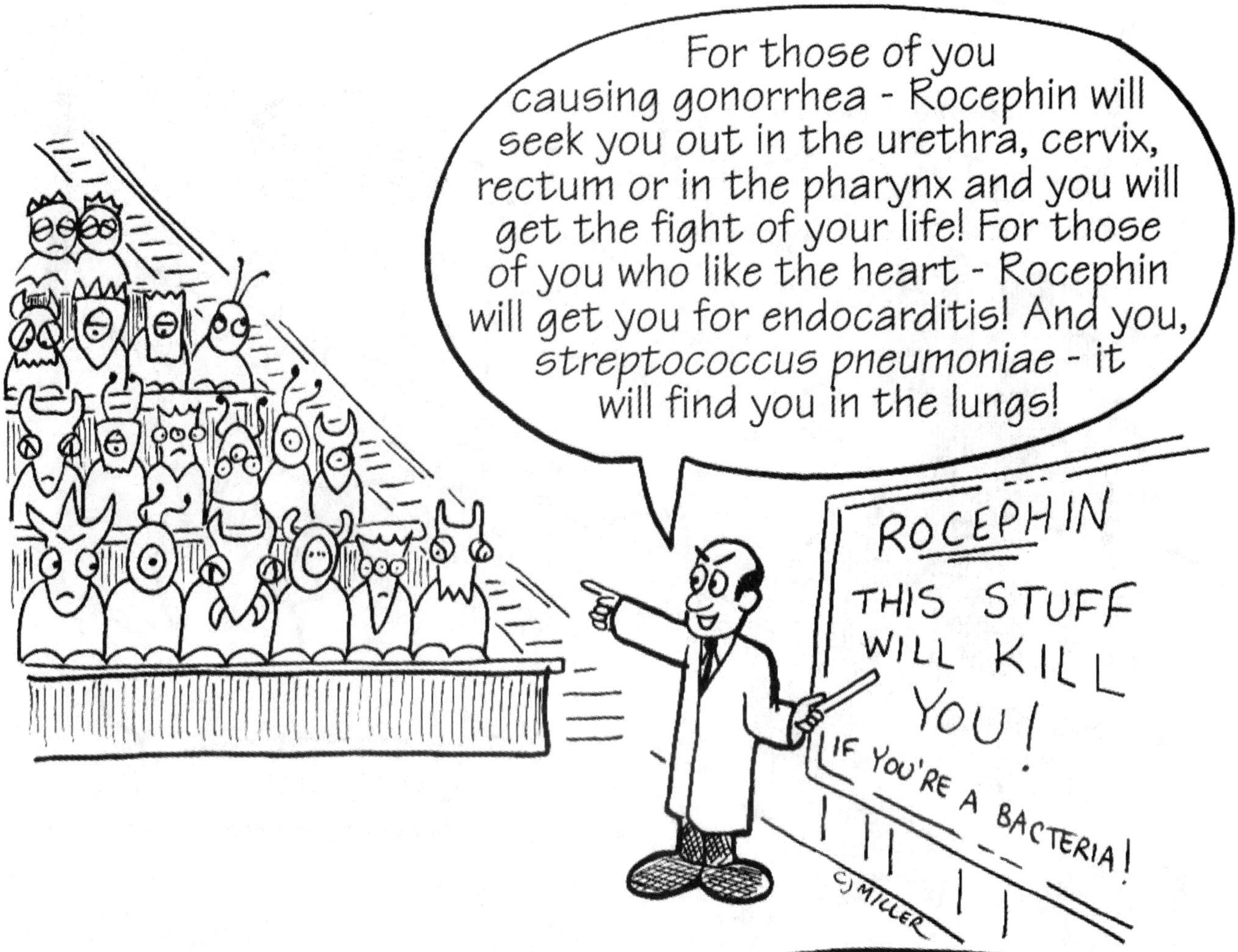
For those of you causing gonorrhea - Rocephin will seek you out in the urethra, cervix, rectum or in the pharynx and you will get the fight of your life! For those of you who like the heart - Rocephin will get you for endocarditis! And you, *streptococcus pneumoniae* - it will find you in the lungs!
ROCEPHIN
THIS STUFF WILL KILL YOU!
IF YOU'RE A BACTERIA!
©J MILLER

Caution:
Renal and hepatic impairment
History of ulcerative colitis
Concurrent use with nephrotoxic medications

Contraindication:
History of allergy to penicillins or cephalosporins.

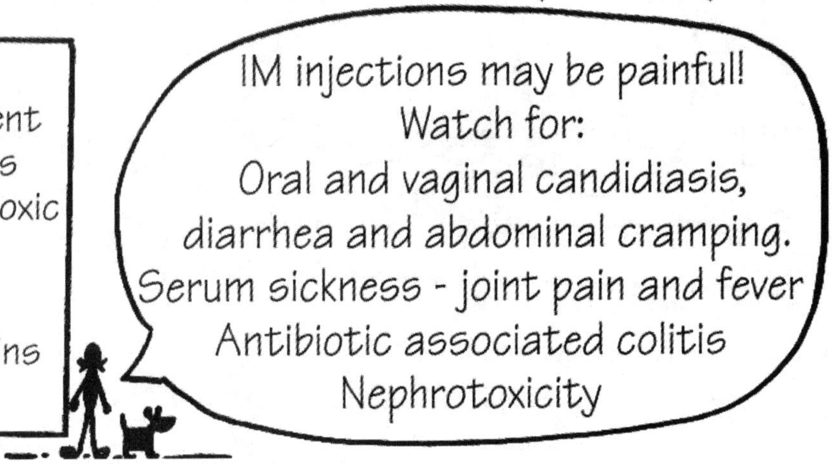
IM injections may be painful!
Watch for:
Oral and vaginal candidiasis, diarrhea and abdominal cramping.
Serum sickness - joint pain and fever
Antibiotic associated colitis
Nephrotoxicity

Cephalosporins

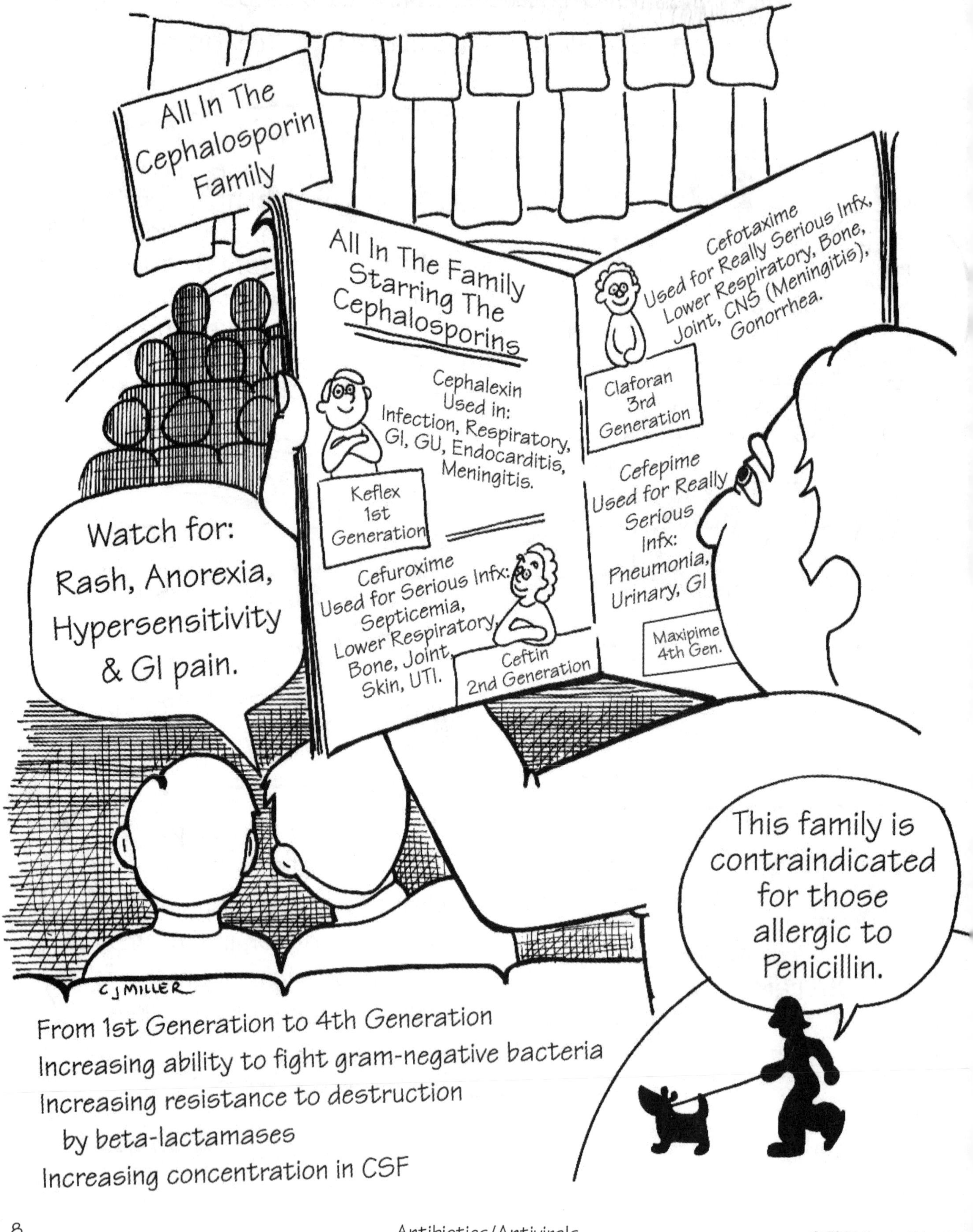
All In The Cephalosporin Family
All In The Family Starring The Cephalosporins
Cephalexin Used in: Infection, Respiratory, GI, GU, Endocarditis, Meningitis.
Keflex 1st Generation
Cefuroxime Used for Serious Infx: Septicemia, Lower Respiratory, Bone, Joint, Skin, UTI.
Ceftin 2nd Generation
Cefotaxime Used for Really Serious Infx, Lower Respiratory, Bone, Joint, CNS (Meningitis), Gonorrhea.
Claforan 3rd Generation
Cefepime Used for Really Serious Infx: Pneumonia, Urinary, GI
Maxipime 4th Gen.
Watch for: Rash, Anorexia, Hypersensitivity & GI pain.
This family is contraindicated for those allergic to Penicillin.
CJ MILLER

From 1st Generation to 4th Generation
Increasing ability to fight gram-negative bacteria
Increasing resistance to destruction by beta-lactamases
Increasing concentration in CSF

Ciprofloxacin (Cipro)

"For those hard to reach chronic bacterial infections"

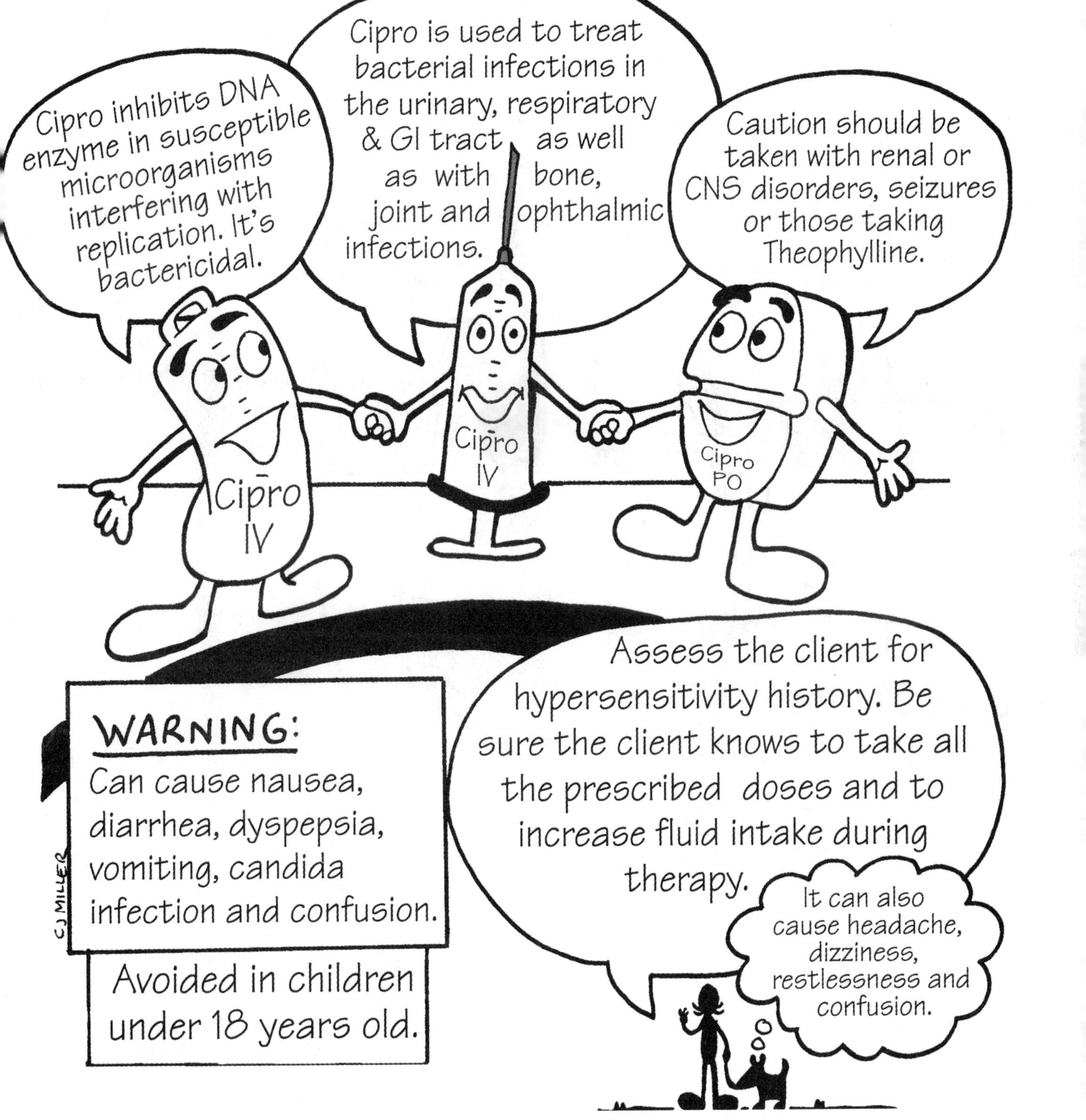
Cipro inhibits DNA enzyme in susceptible microorganisms interfering with replication. It's bactericidal.
Cipro is used to treat bacterial infections in the urinary, respiratory & GI tract as well as with bone, joint and ophthalmic infections.
Caution should be taken with renal or CNS disorders, seizures or those taking Theophylline.
Cipro IV
Cipro IV
Cipro PO
WARNING: Can cause nausea, diarrhea, dyspepsia, vomiting, candida infection and confusion.
Avoided in children under 18 years old.
Assess the client for hypersensitivity history. Be sure the client knows to take all the prescribed doses and to increase fluid intake during therapy.
It can also cause headache, dizziness, restlessness and confusion.
C J MILLER

Gatifloxacin (Tequin)

"Tequin for Acute Bacterial Exacerbations"

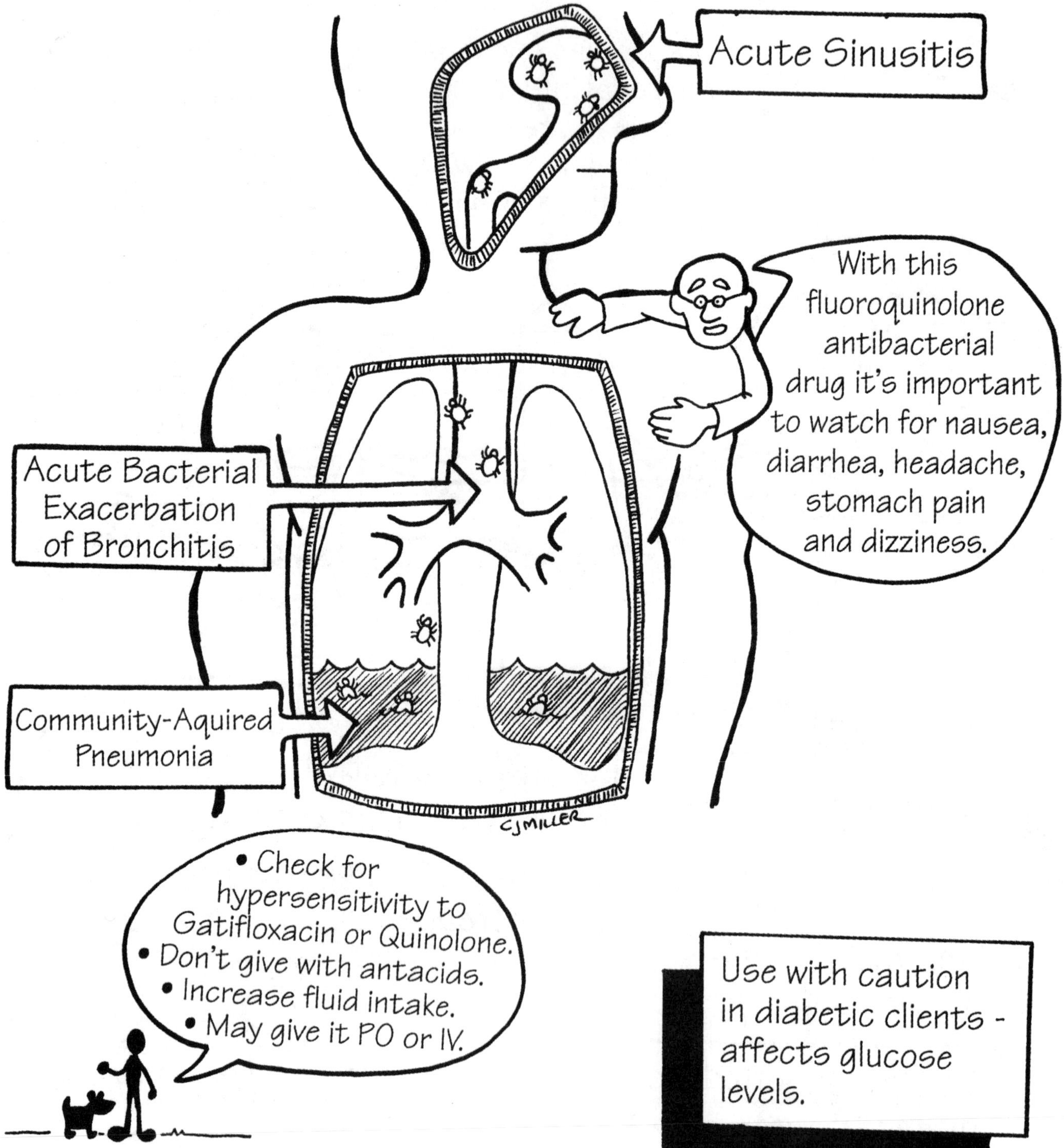

Acute Sinusitis
With this fluoroquinolone antibacterial drug it's important to watch for nausea, diarrhea, headache, stomach pain and dizziness.
Acute Bacterial Exacerbation of Bronchitis
Community-Aquired Pneumonia
CJMILLER
• Check for hypersensitivity to Gatifloxacin or Quinolone.
• Don't give with antacids.
• Increase fluid intake.
• May give it PO or IV.

Use with caution in diabetic clients - affects glucose levels.

Isoniazide (INH)

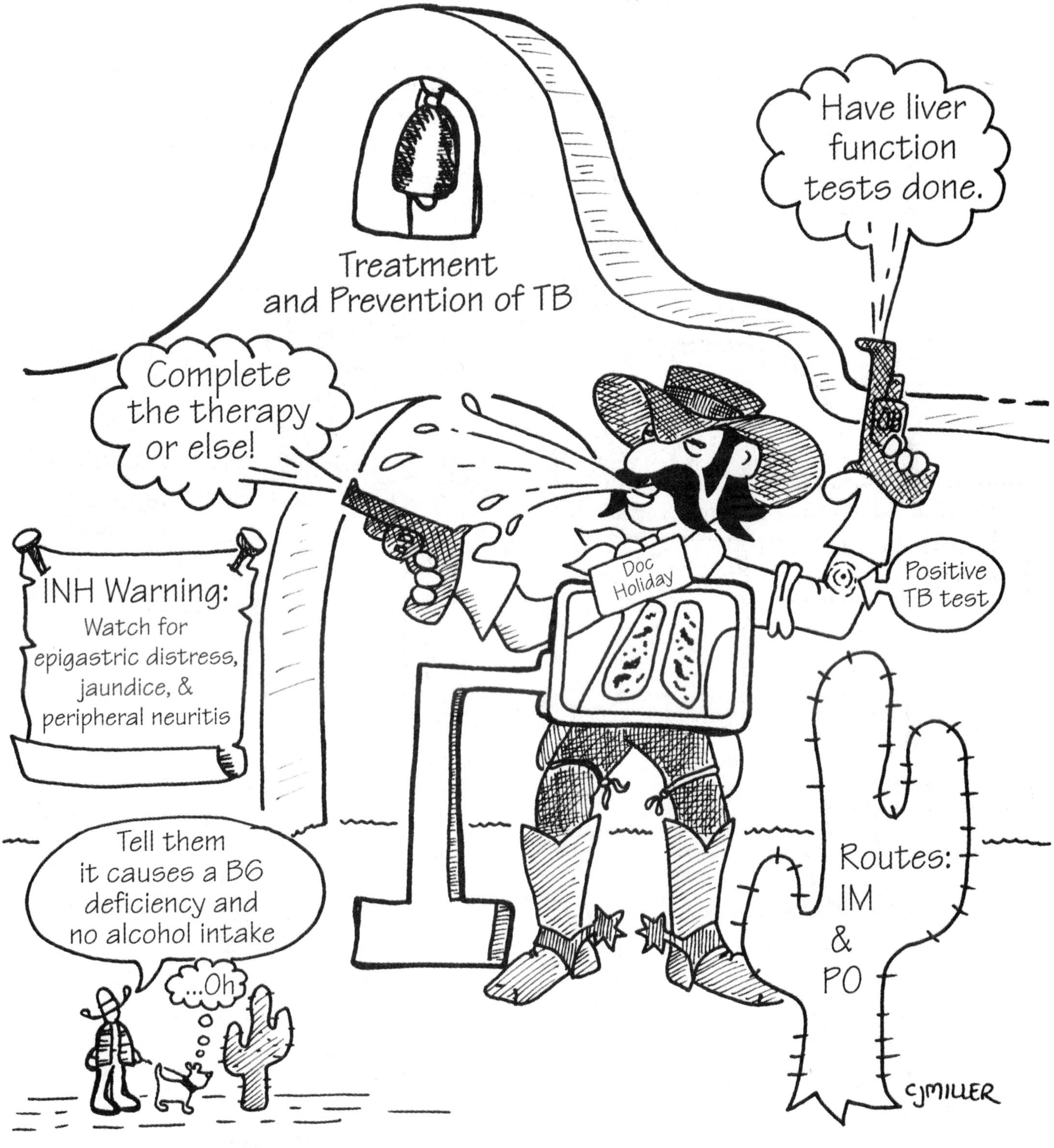

Have liver function tests done.
Treatment and Prevention of TB
Complete the therapy or else!
INH Warning: Watch for epigastric distress, jaundice, & peripheral neuritis
Doc Holiday
Positive TB test
Tell them it causes a B6 deficiency and no alcohol intake
...Oh
Routes: IM & PO
CJMILLER

Metronidazole (Flagyl)

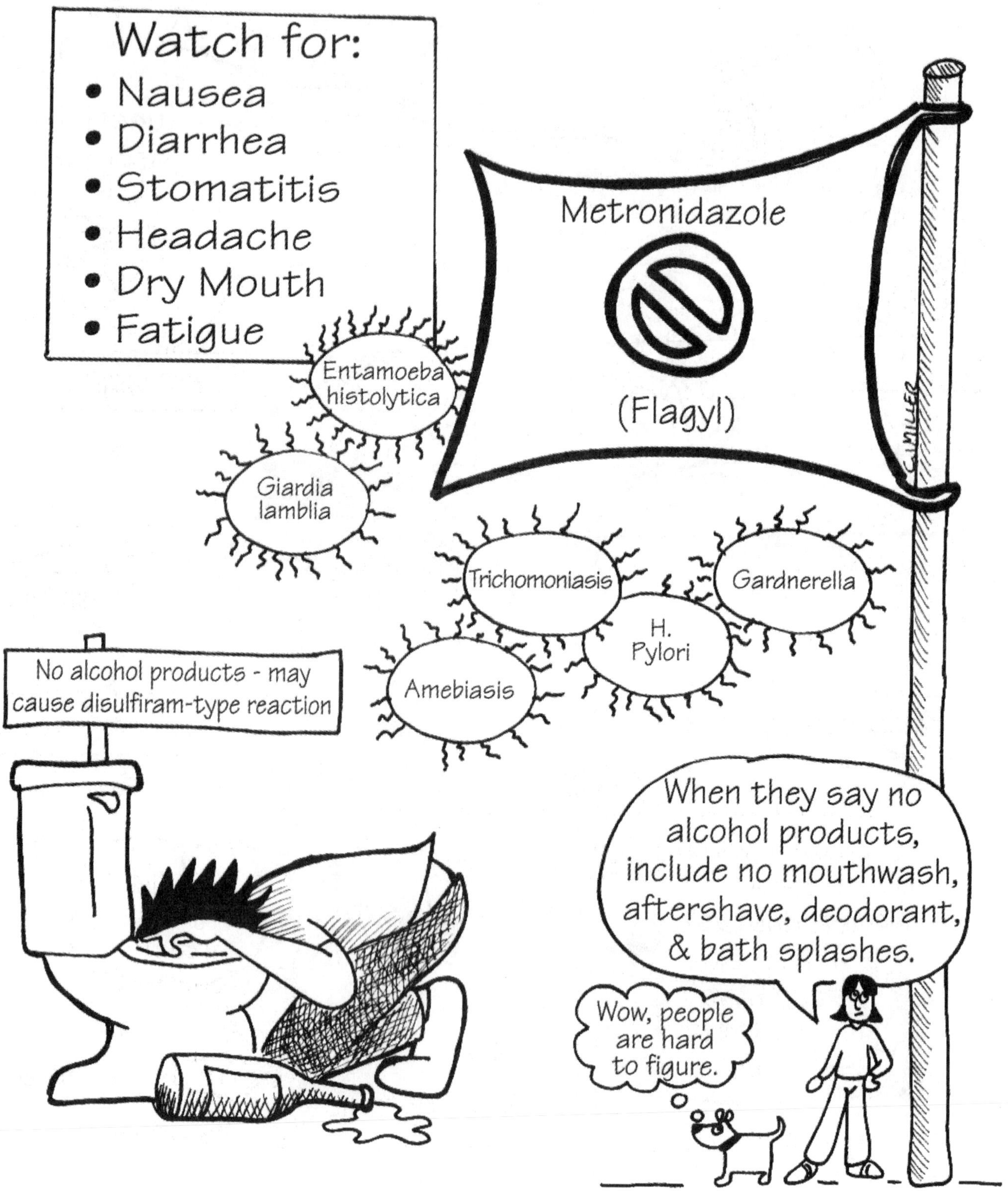

Watch for:
• Nausea
• Diarrhea
• Stomatitis
• Headache
• Dry Mouth
• Fatigue
Metronidazole
(Flagyl)
C. MILLER
Entamoeba histolytica
Giardia lamblia
Trichomoniasis
Gardnerella
H. Pylori
Amebiasis
No alcohol products - may cause disulfiram-type reaction
When they say no alcohol products, include no mouthwash, aftershave, deodorant, & bath splashes.
Wow, people are hard to figure.

Penicillin (PCN)

Uses and Side Effects

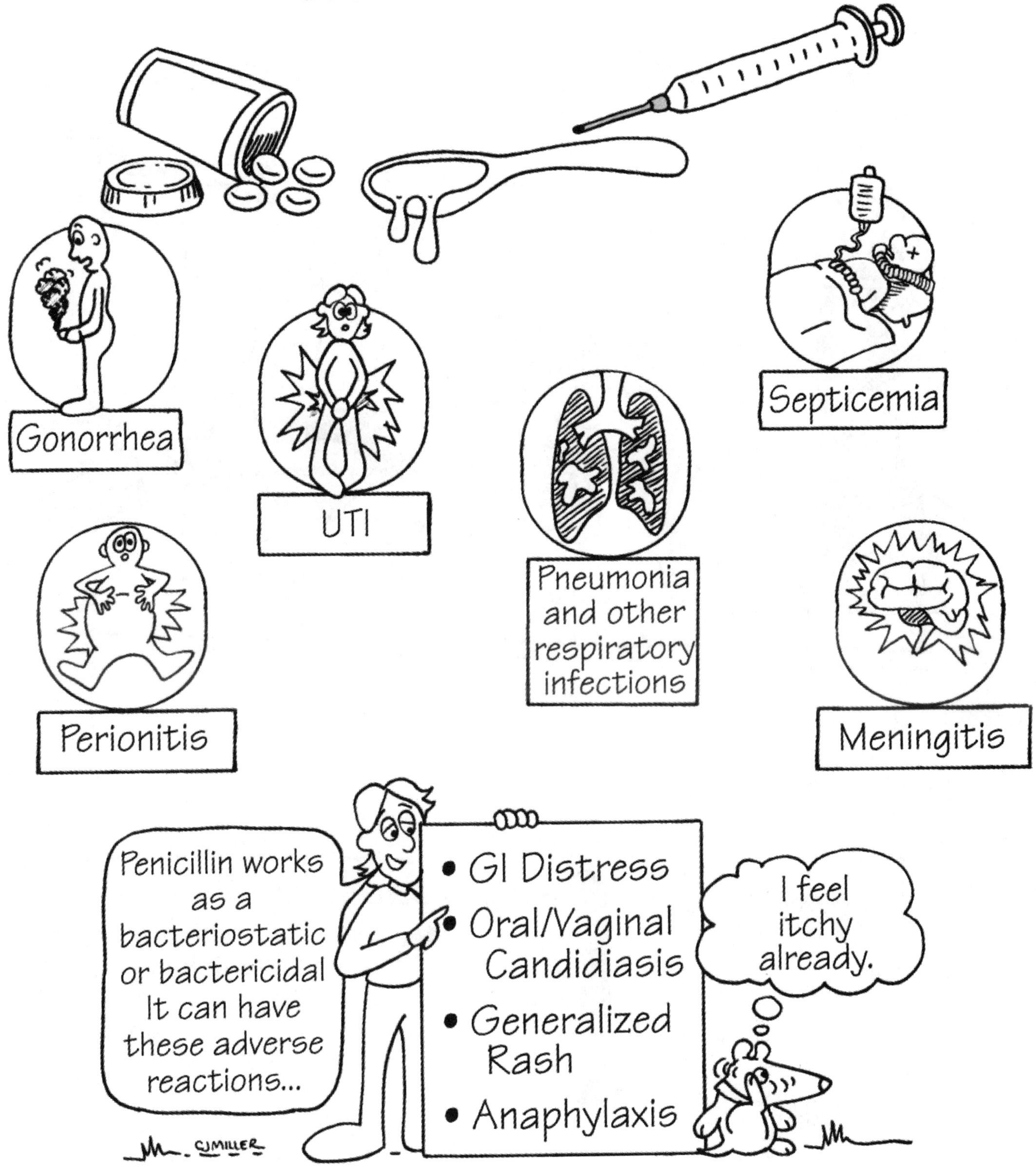

Gonorrhea
UTI
Pneumonia and other respiratory infections
Septicemia
Perionitis
Meningitis
Penicillin works as a bacteriostatic or bactericidal It can have these adverse reactions...
• GI Distress
• Oral/Vaginal Candidiasis
• Generalized Rash
• Anaphylaxis
I feel itchy already.
CJMILLER

Tetracycline Uses

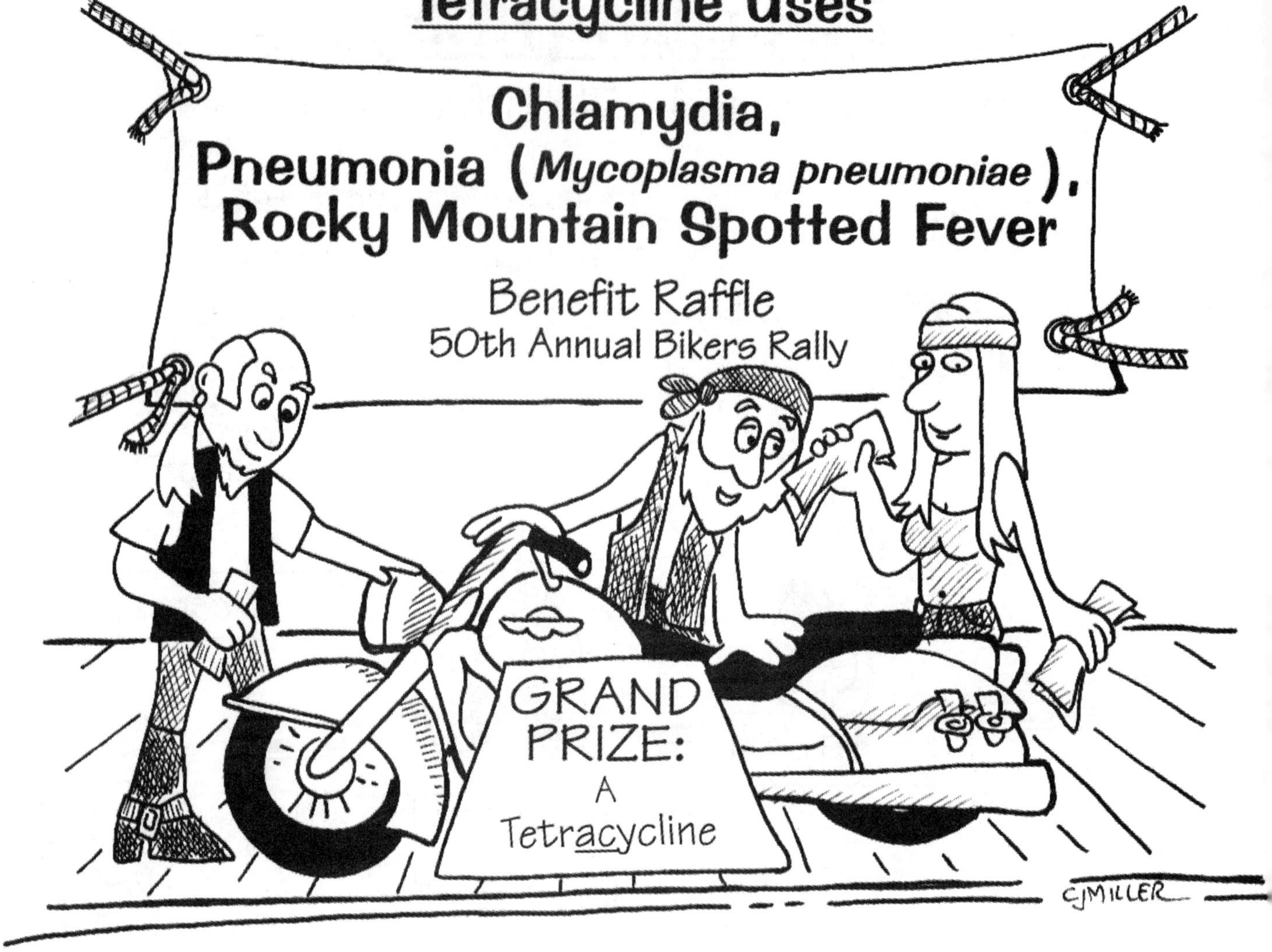
Chlamydia,
Pneumonia (*Mycoplasma pneumoniae*),
Rocky Mountain Spotted Fever
Benefit Raffle
50th Annual Bikers Rally
GRAND PRIZE:
A
Tetracycline
CJMILLER

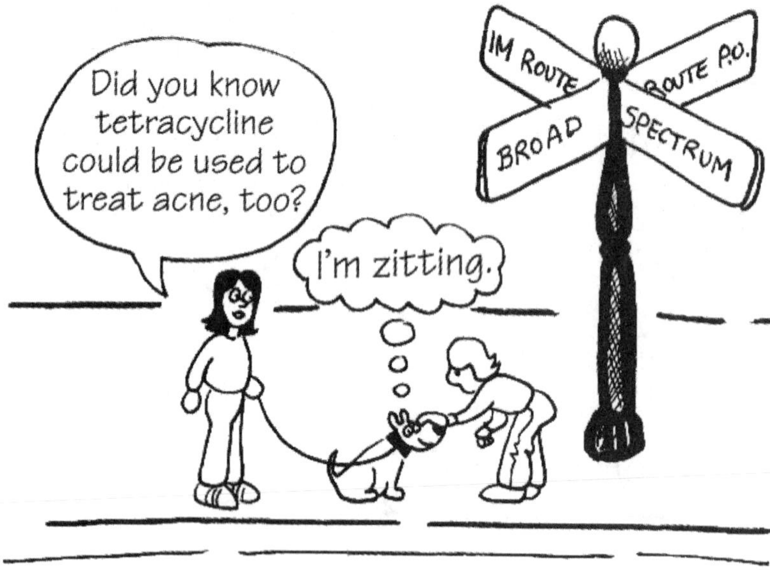
Did you know tetracycline could be used to treat acne, too?
I'm zitting.
IM ROUTE
ROUTE P.O.
BROAD
SPECTRUM

Caution:

- Staining of deciduous teeth if taken after 4th month of pregnancy.
- Staining of permanent teeth if taken from ages 4 months to 8 years.
- Don't give with milk, calcium supplements, or antacids.

Chlorambucil (Leukeran)

"Abnormal cell growth called Lymphocytic Leukemia, Non-Hodgkin's and Hodgkin's Disease"

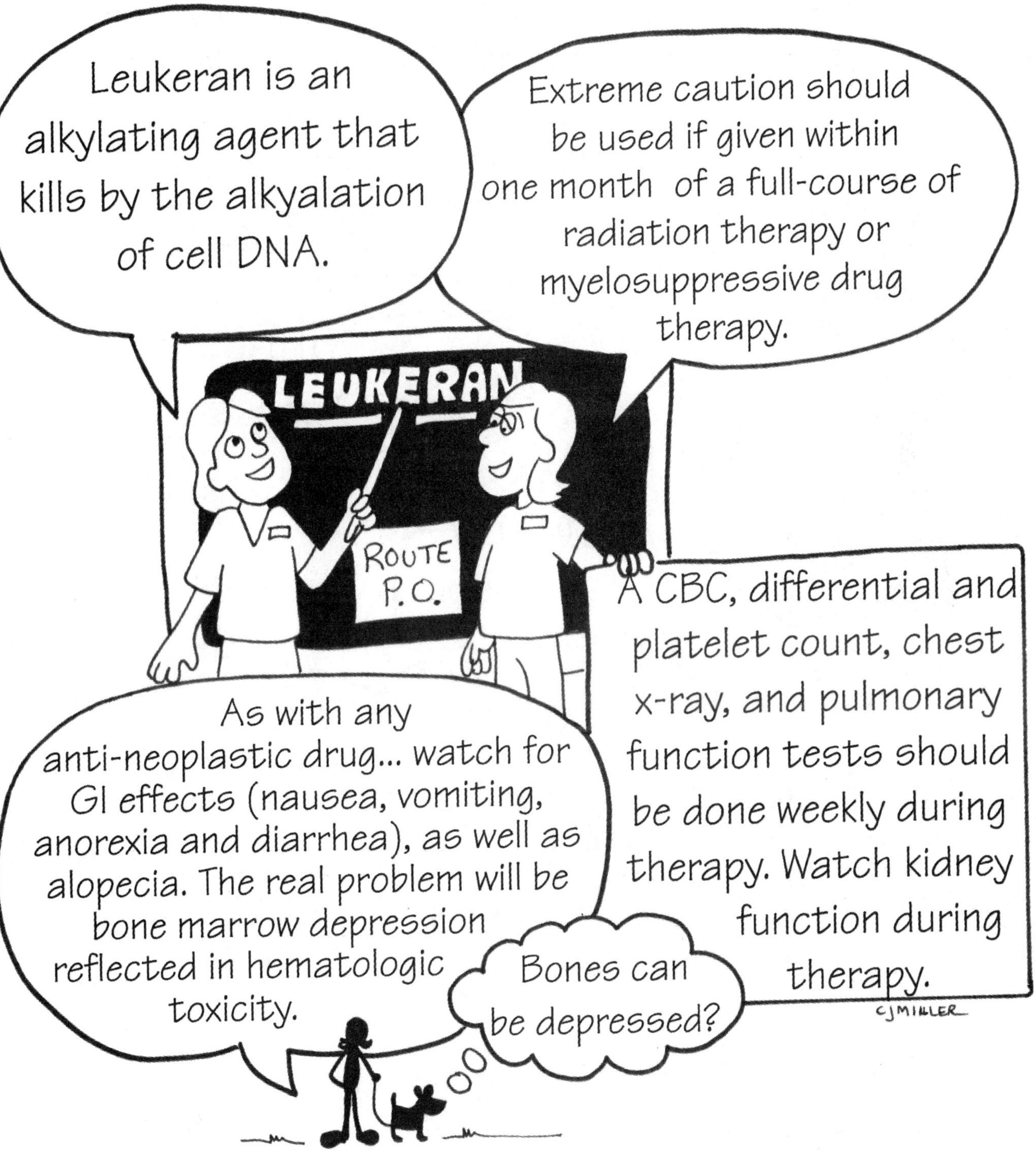

Leukeran is an alkylating agent that kills by the alkyalation of cell DNA.
Extreme caution should be used if given within one month of a full-course of radiation therapy or myelosuppressive drug therapy.
LEUKERAN
ROUTE P.O.
A CBC, differential and platelet count, chest x-ray, and pulmonary function tests should be done weekly during therapy. Watch kidney function during therapy.
As with any anti-neoplastic drug... watch for GI effects (nausea, vomiting, anorexia and diarrhea), as well as alopecia. The real problem will be bone marrow depression reflected in hematologic toxicity.
Bones can be depressed?
CJMILLER

ACE Inhibitors

Angiotensin - Converting Enzyme

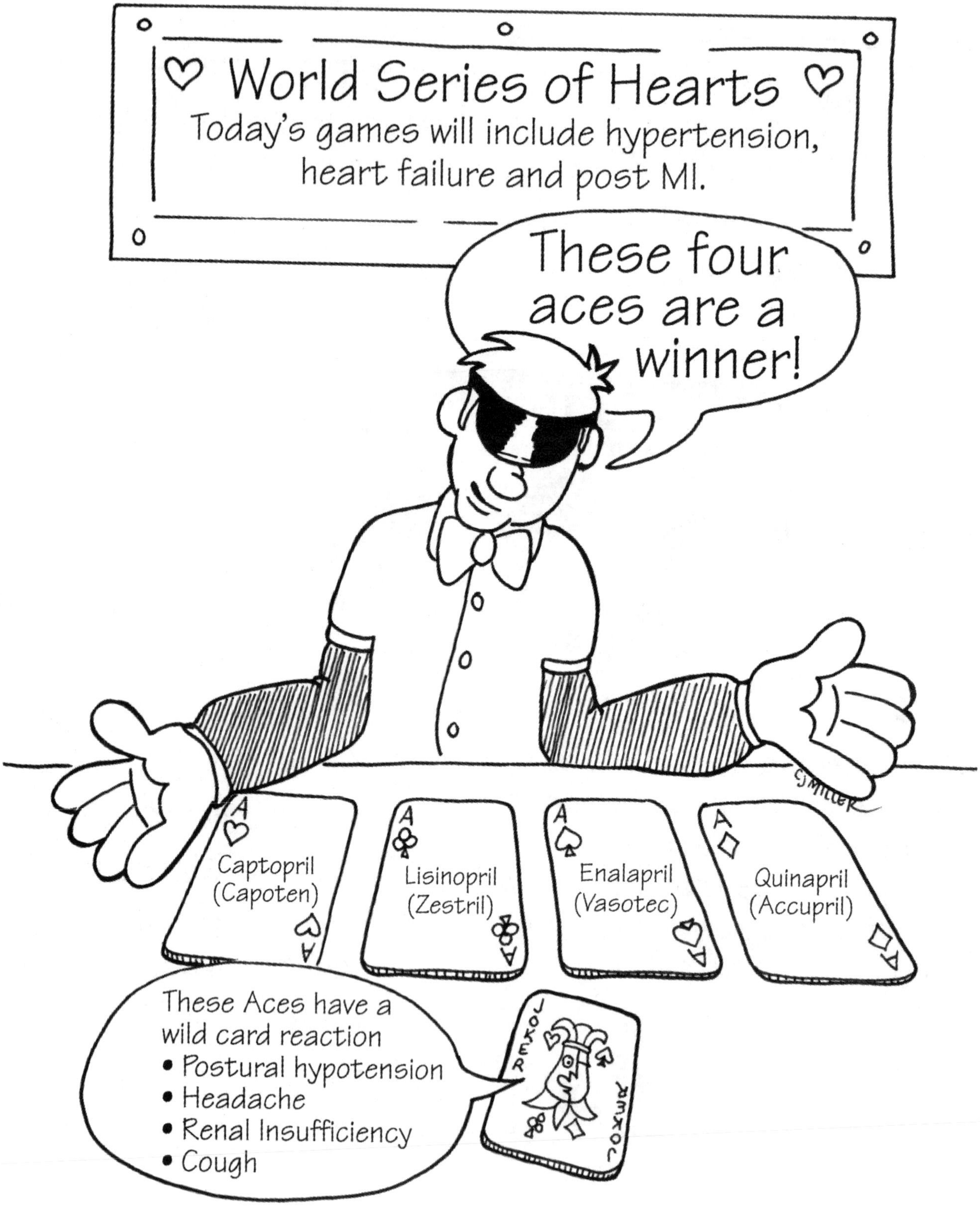

World Series of Hearts
Today's games will include hypertension, heart failure and post MI.
These four aces are a winner!
Captopril (Capoten)
Lisinopril (Zestril)
Enalapril (Vasotec)
Quinapril (Accupril)
These Aces have a wild card reaction
• Postural hypotension
• Headache
• Renal Insufficiency
• Cough
JOKER

Amiodarone (Cordarone)

"Don Cordarone... The Enforcer"

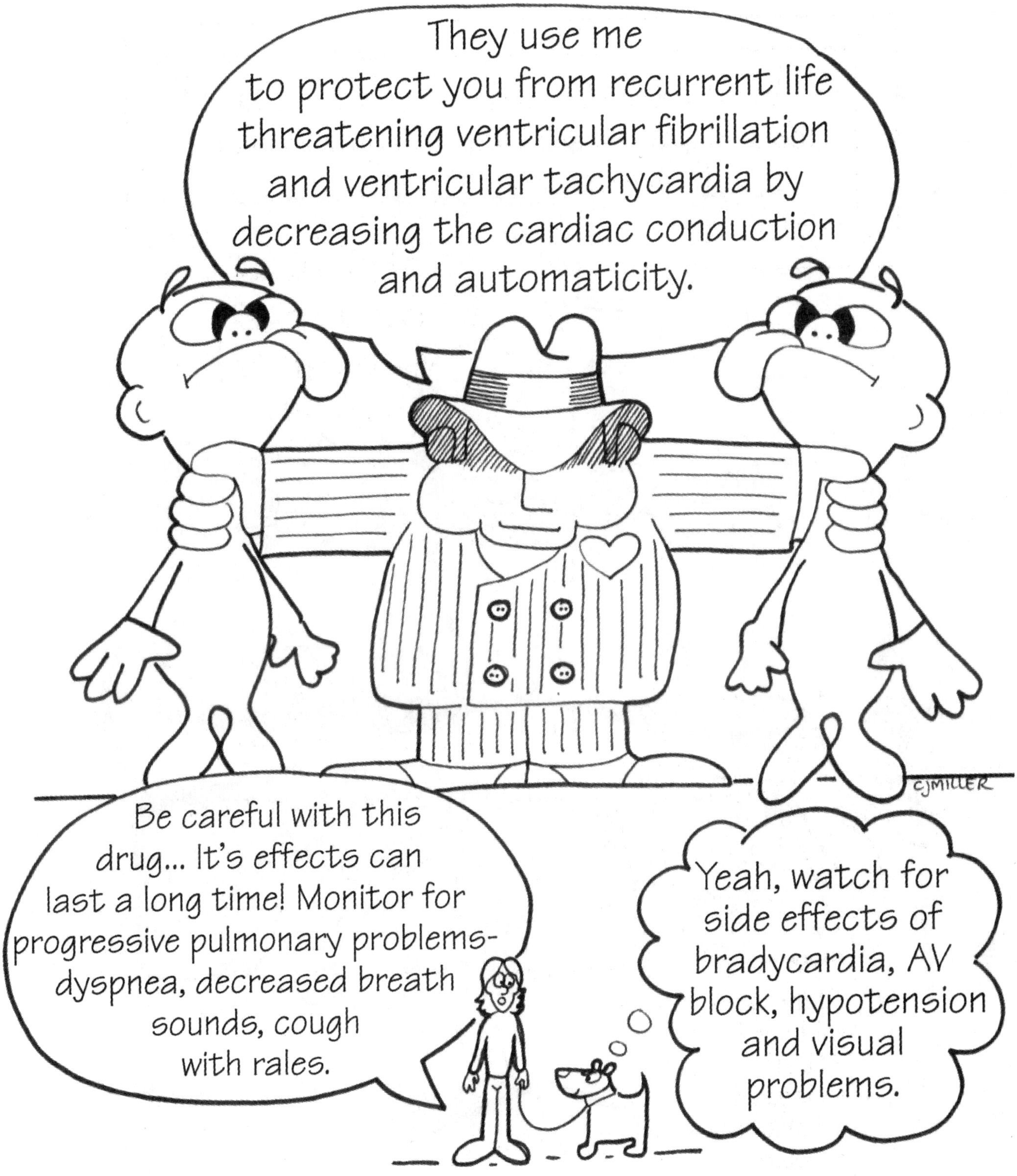
They use me to protect you from recurrent life threatening ventricular fibrillation and ventricular tachycardia by decreasing the cardiac conduction and automaticity.
CJMILLER
Be careful with this drug... It's effects can last a long time! Monitor for progressive pulmonary problems- dyspnea, decreased breath sounds, cough with rales.
Yeah, watch for side effects of bradycardia, AV block, hypotension and visual problems.

Antidysrhythmics

THE ANTIDYSRHYTHMIC SCHOOL OF DANCE
If you've got good rhythm, you can dance to any beat
Dance Night
Sponsored by
The Faculty
We've Got The Rhythm
Diltiazem (Cardizem)
Propranolol (Inderal)
Quinidine Sulfate (Novoquindin)
Amiodarone (Cordarone)
Watch for:
Bradycardia, headache, edema of feet & legs, dizziness
Hypotension, bradycardia, bronchospasm
Headache, bradycardia, diarrhea & immunologic reaction
Pulmonary toxicity, visual impairment, bradycardia, hypotension
CJMILLER

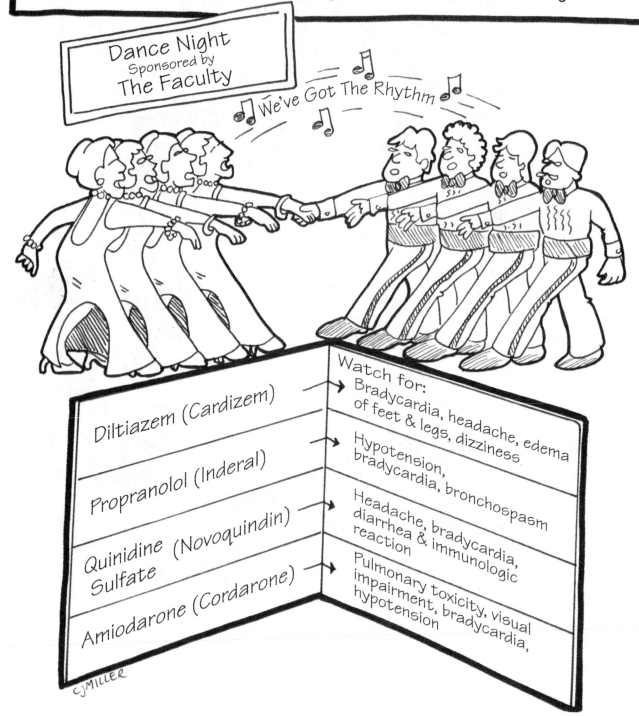

Antihypertensives

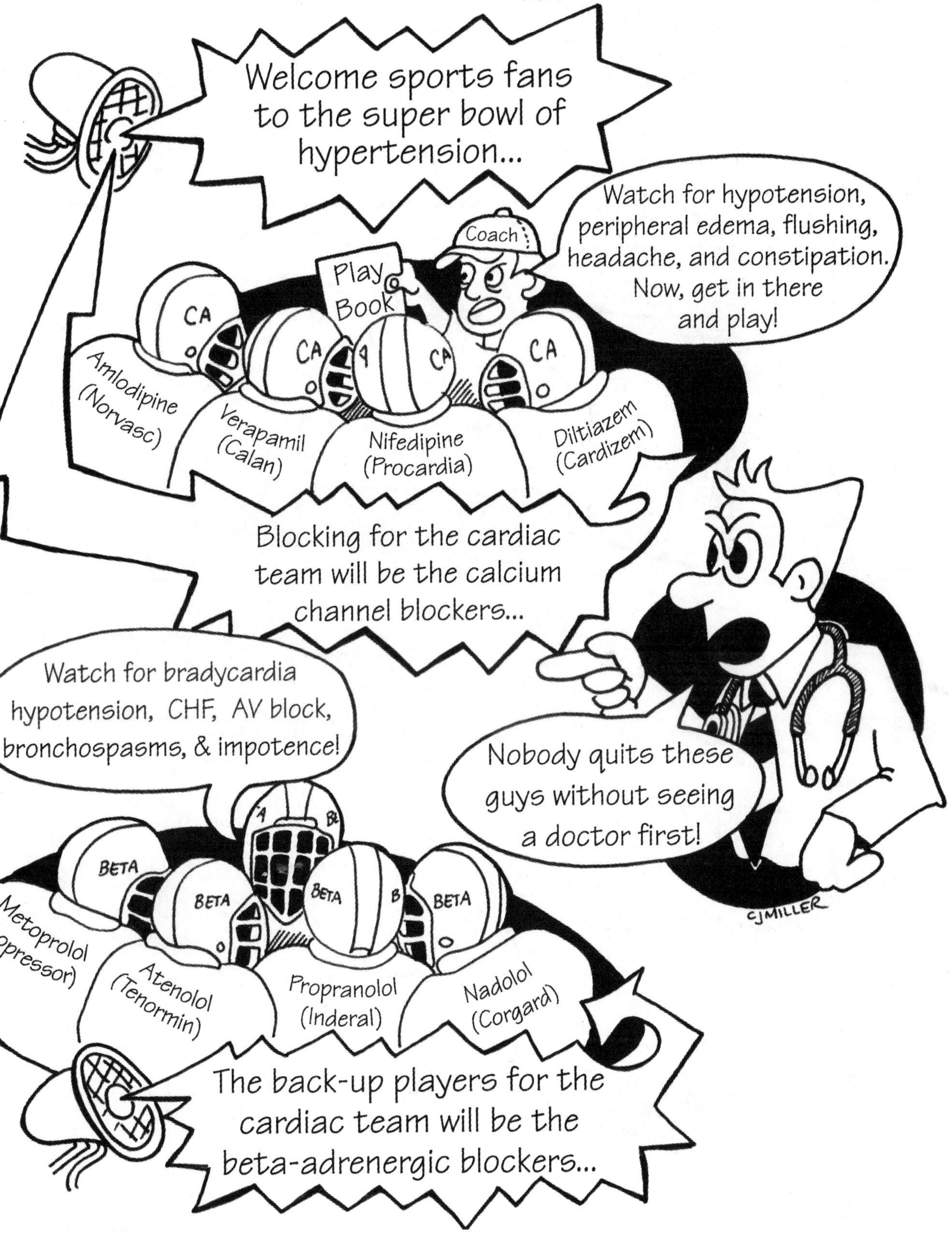

Welcome sports fans to the super bowl of hypertension...
Coach
Play Book
Watch for hypotension, peripheral edema, flushing, headache, and constipation. Now, get in there and play!
CA
CA
CA
CA
Amlodipine (Norvasc)
Verapamil (Calan)
Nifedipine (Procardia)
Diltiazem (Cardizem)
Blocking for the cardiac team will be the calcium channel blockers...
Watch for bradycardia hypotension, CHF, AV block, bronchospasms, & impotence!
Nobody quits these guys without seeing a doctor first!
BETA
BETA
BETA
BETA
Metoprolol (Lopressor)
Atenolol (Tenormin)
Propranolol (Inderal)
Nadolol (Corgard)
CJMILLER
The back-up players for the cardiac team will be the beta-adrenergic blockers...

Cholestyramine Resin (Questran)

"Separating the Good From the Bad"

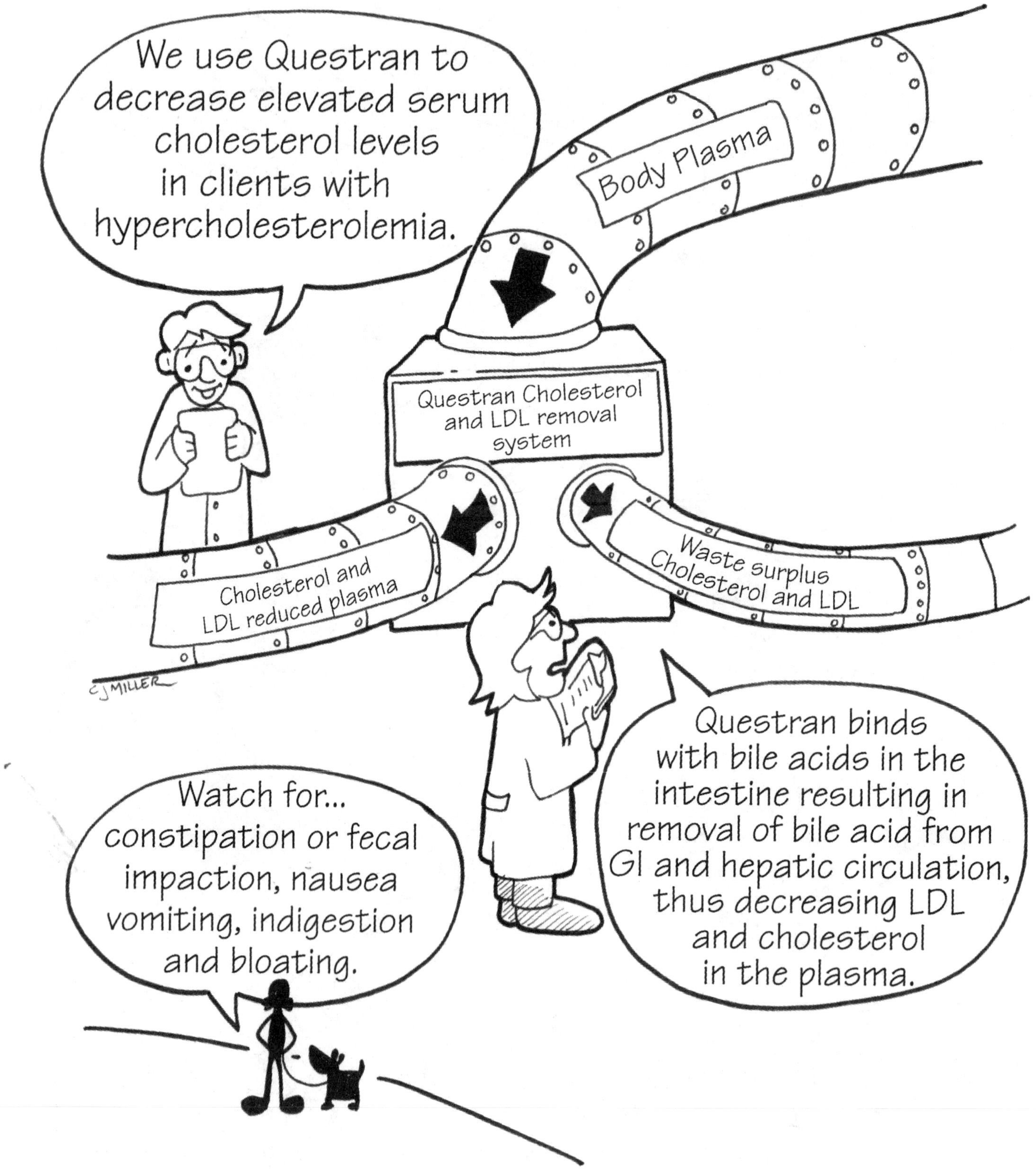
We use Questran to decrease elevated serum cholesterol levels in clients with hypercholesterolemia.
Body Plasma
Questran Cholesterol and LDL removal system
Cholesterol and LDL reduced plasma
Waste surplus Cholesterol and LDL
CJ MILLER
Questran binds with bile acids in the intestine resulting in removal of bile acid from GI and hepatic circulation, thus decreasing LDL and cholesterol in the plasma.
Watch for... constipation or fecal impaction, nausea vomiting, indigestion and bloating.

Digitalis

The Wizard of Digitalis

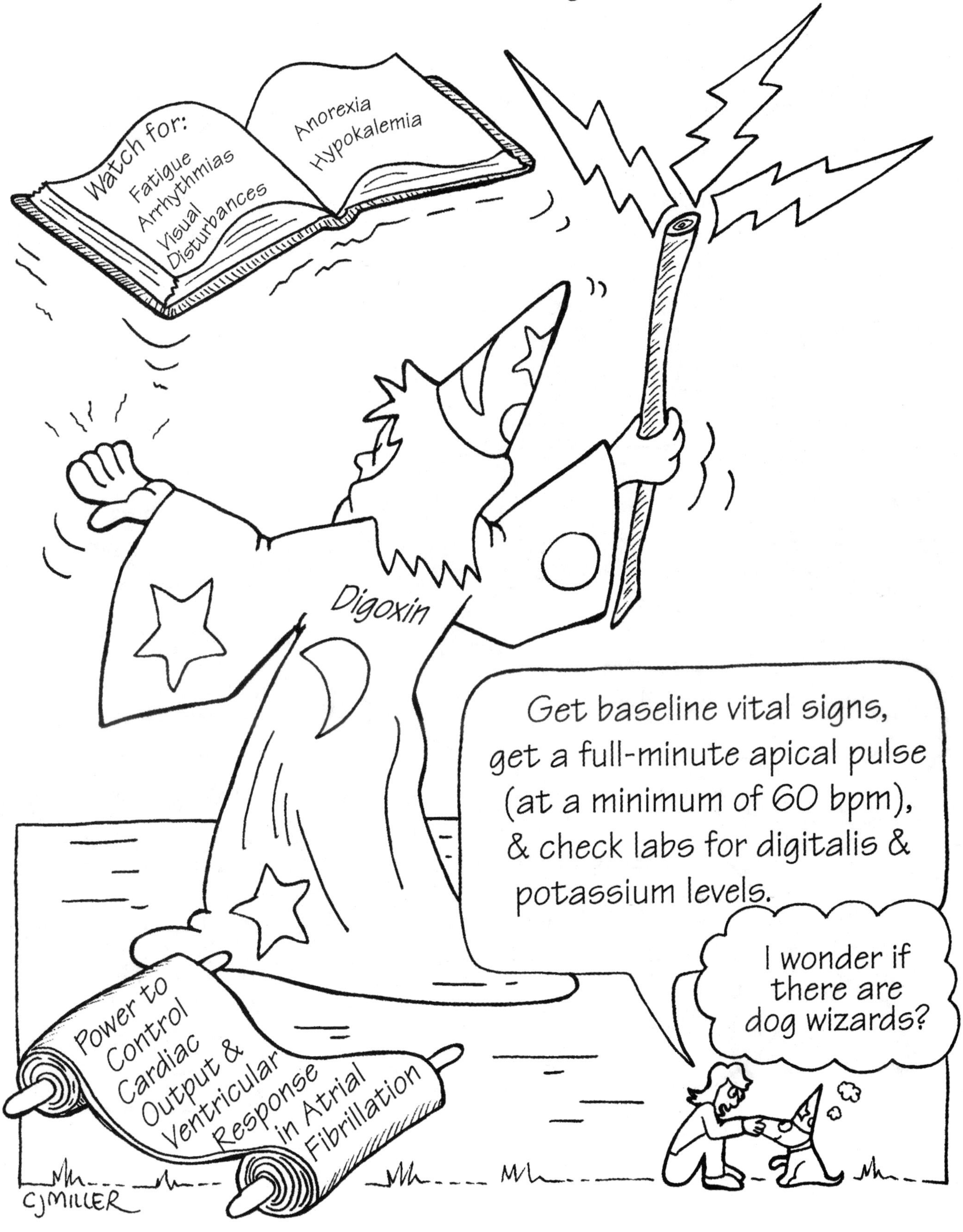

Watch for:
Fatigue
Arrhythmias
Visual Disturbances
Anorexia
Hypokalemia
Digoxin
Get baseline vital signs, get a full-minute apical pulse (at a minimum of 60 bpm), & check labs for digitalis & potassium levels.
I wonder if there are dog wizards?
Power to Control Cardiac Output & Ventricular Response in Atrial Fibrillation
CJMILLER

Fosinopril (Monopril)

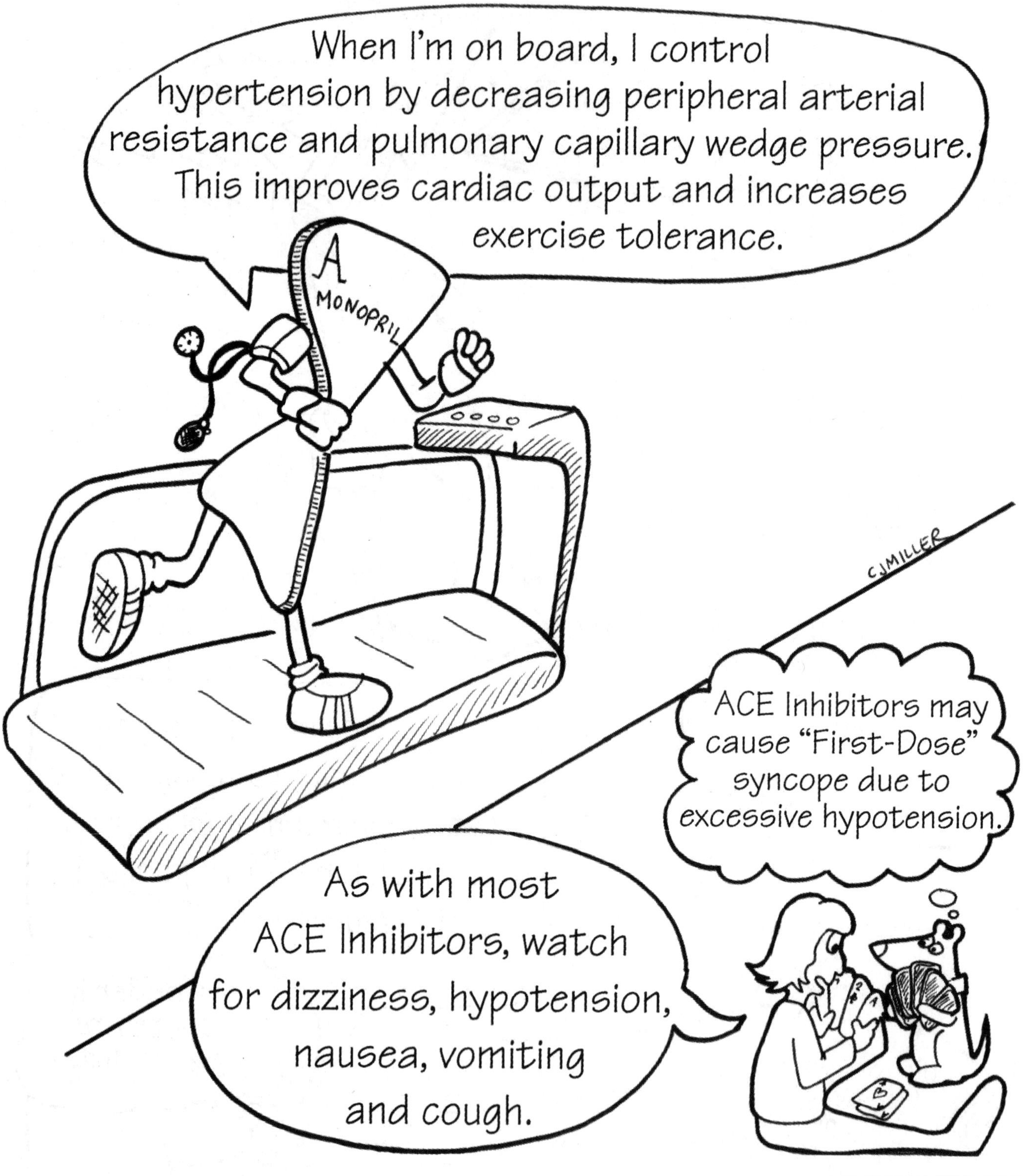

When I'm on board, I control hypertension by decreasing peripheral arterial resistance and pulmonary capillary wedge pressure. This improves cardiac output and increases exercise tolerance.
A
MONOPRIL
CJMILLER
ACE Inhibitors may cause "First-Dose" syncope due to excessive hypotension.
As with most ACE Inhibitors, watch for dizziness, hypotension, nausea, vomiting and cough.

Gemfibrozil (Lopid)

"If it tastes good, it's probably bad for you."

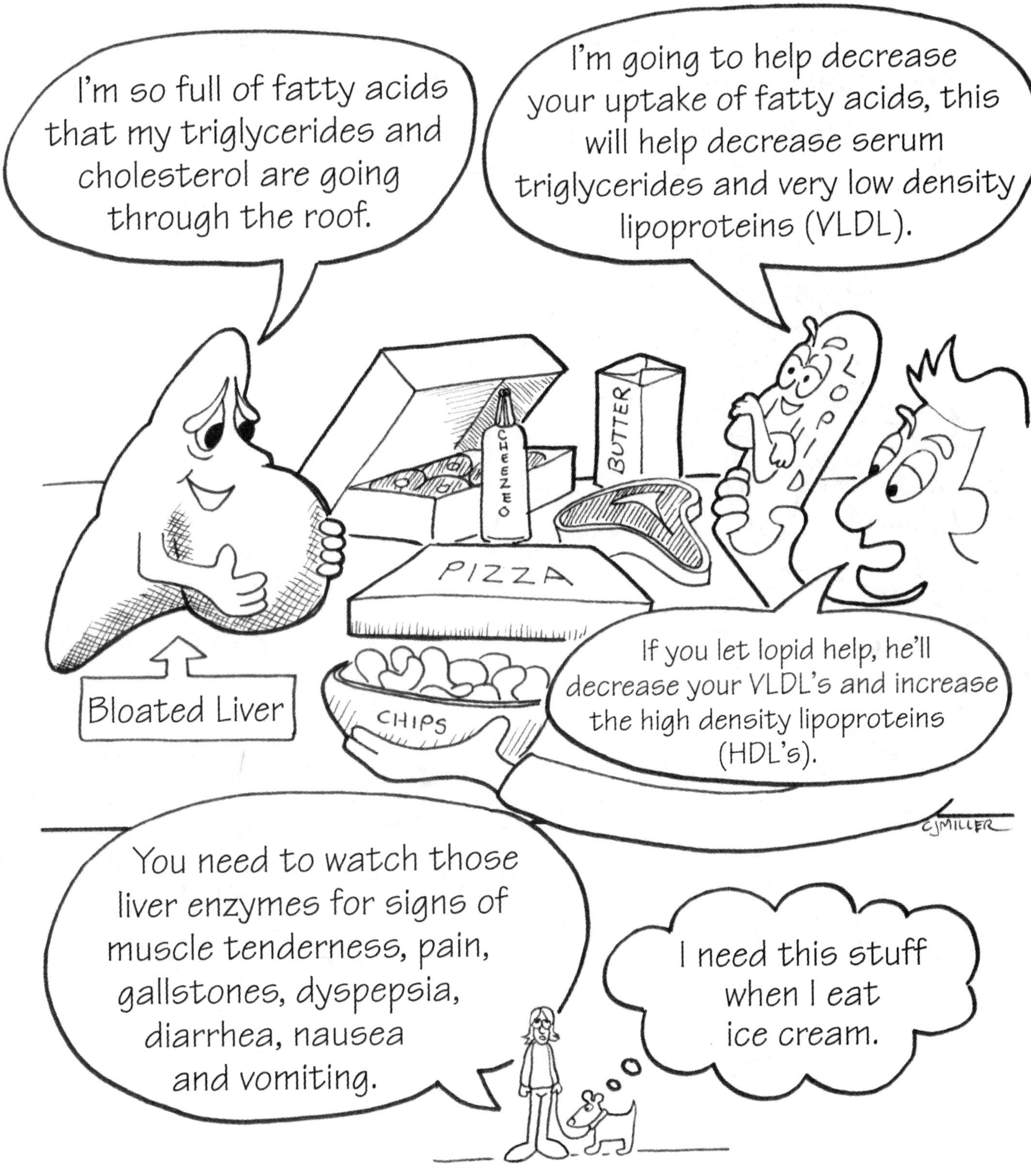
I'm so full of fatty acids that my triglycerides and cholesterol are going through the roof.
I'm going to help decrease your uptake of fatty acids, this will help decrease serum triglycerides and very low density lipoproteins (VLDL).
LOPID
BUTTER
CHEEZO
PIZZA
CHIPS
Bloated Liver
If you let lopid help, he'll decrease your VLDL's and increase the high density lipoproteins (HDL's).
CJMILLER
You need to watch those liver enzymes for signs of muscle tenderness, pain, gallstones, dyspepsia, diarrhea, nausea and vomiting.
I need this stuff when I eat ice cream.

Nitroglycerin

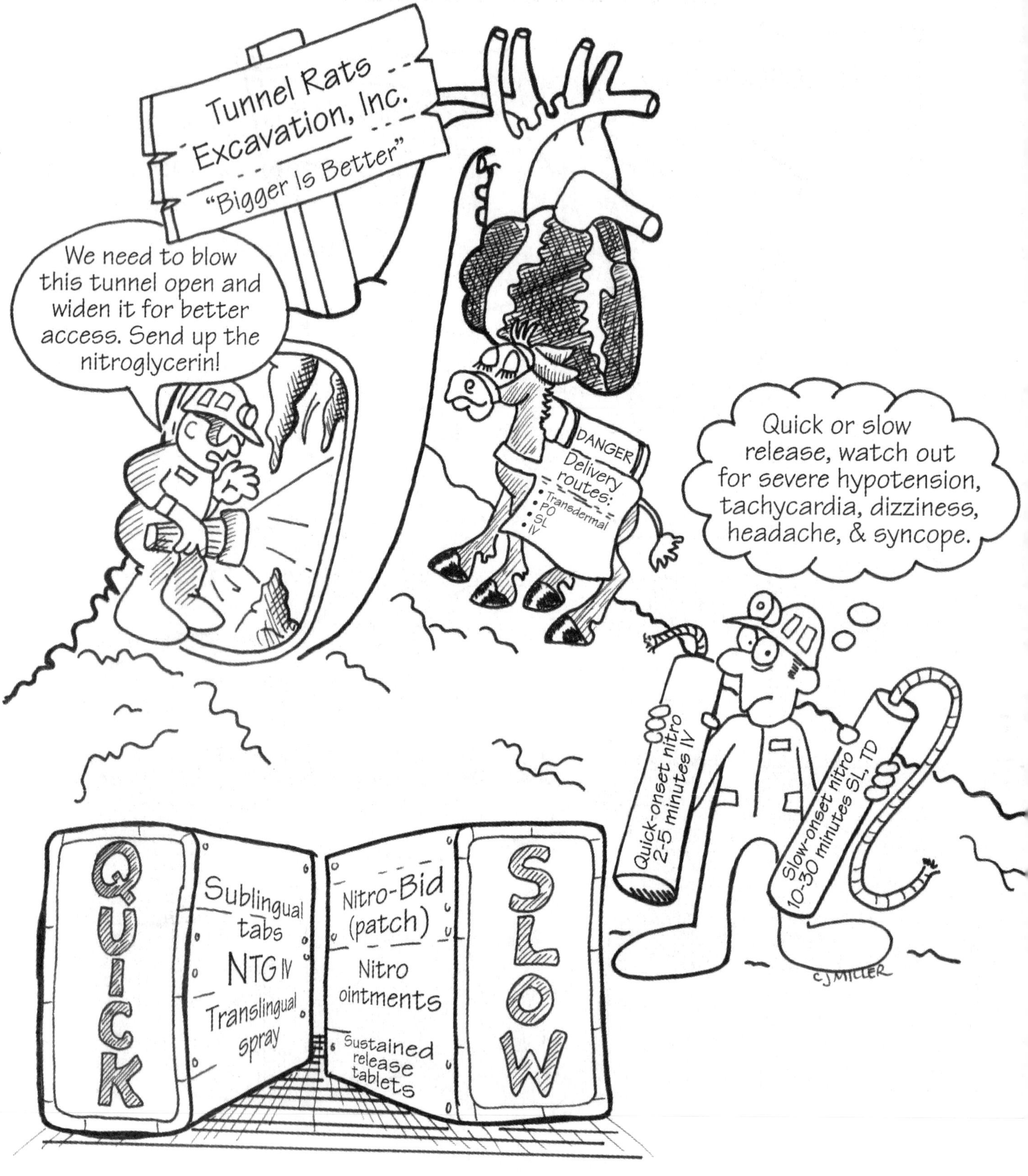
Tunnel Rats Excavation, Inc.
"Bigger Is Better"
We need to blow this tunnel open and widen it for better access. Send up the nitroglycerin!
DANGER
Delivery routes:
• Transdermal
• PO
• SL
• IV
Quick or slow release, watch out for severe hypotension, tachycardia, dizziness, headache, & syncope.
Quick-onset nitro 2-5 minutes IV
Slow-onset nitro 10-30 minutes SL, TD
QUICK
Sublingual tabs
NTG IV
Translingual spray
SLOW
Nitro-Bid (patch)
Nitro ointments
Sustained release tablets
CJ MILLER

Antihistamines

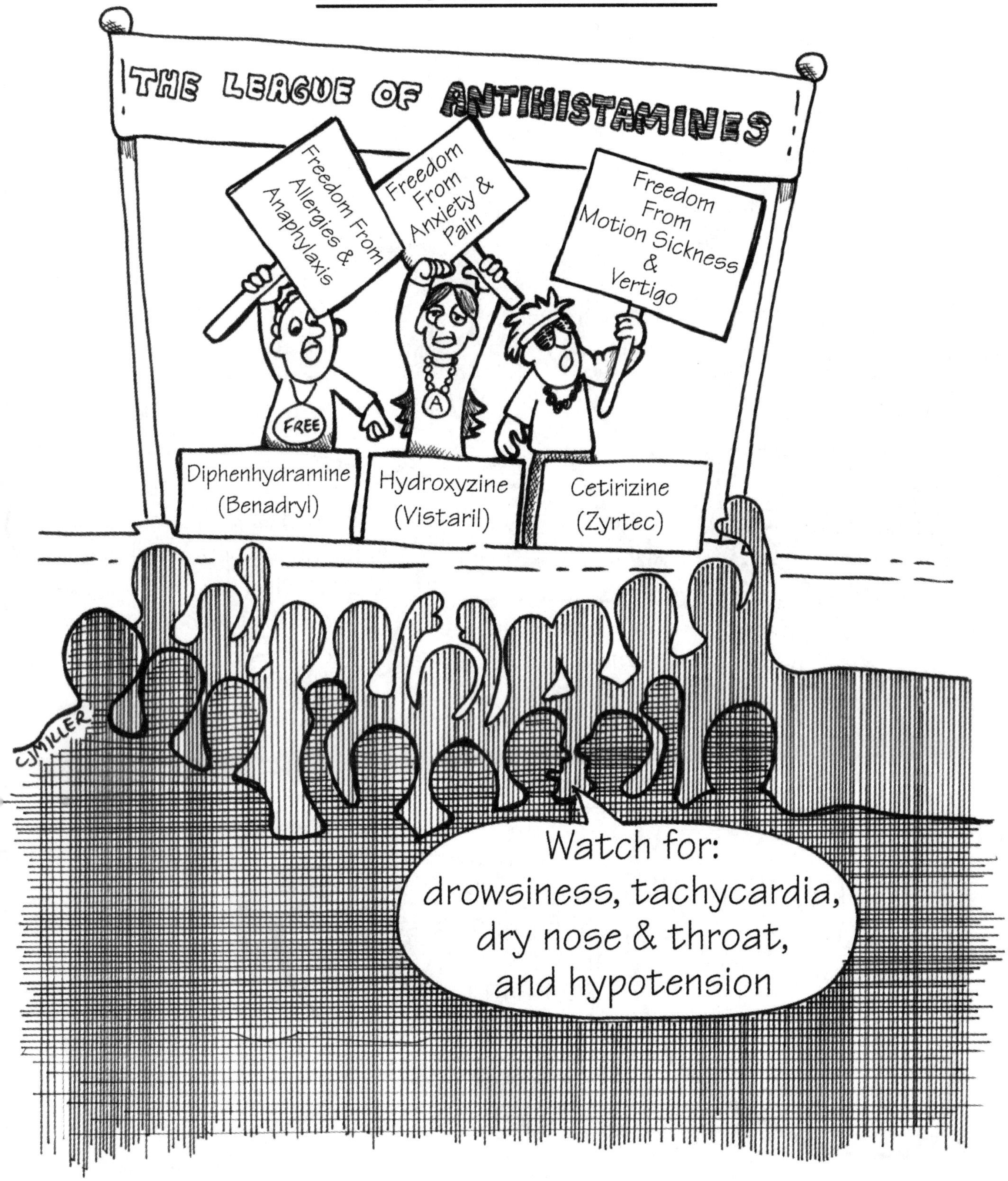

Antitussives, Expectorants, & Mucolytics

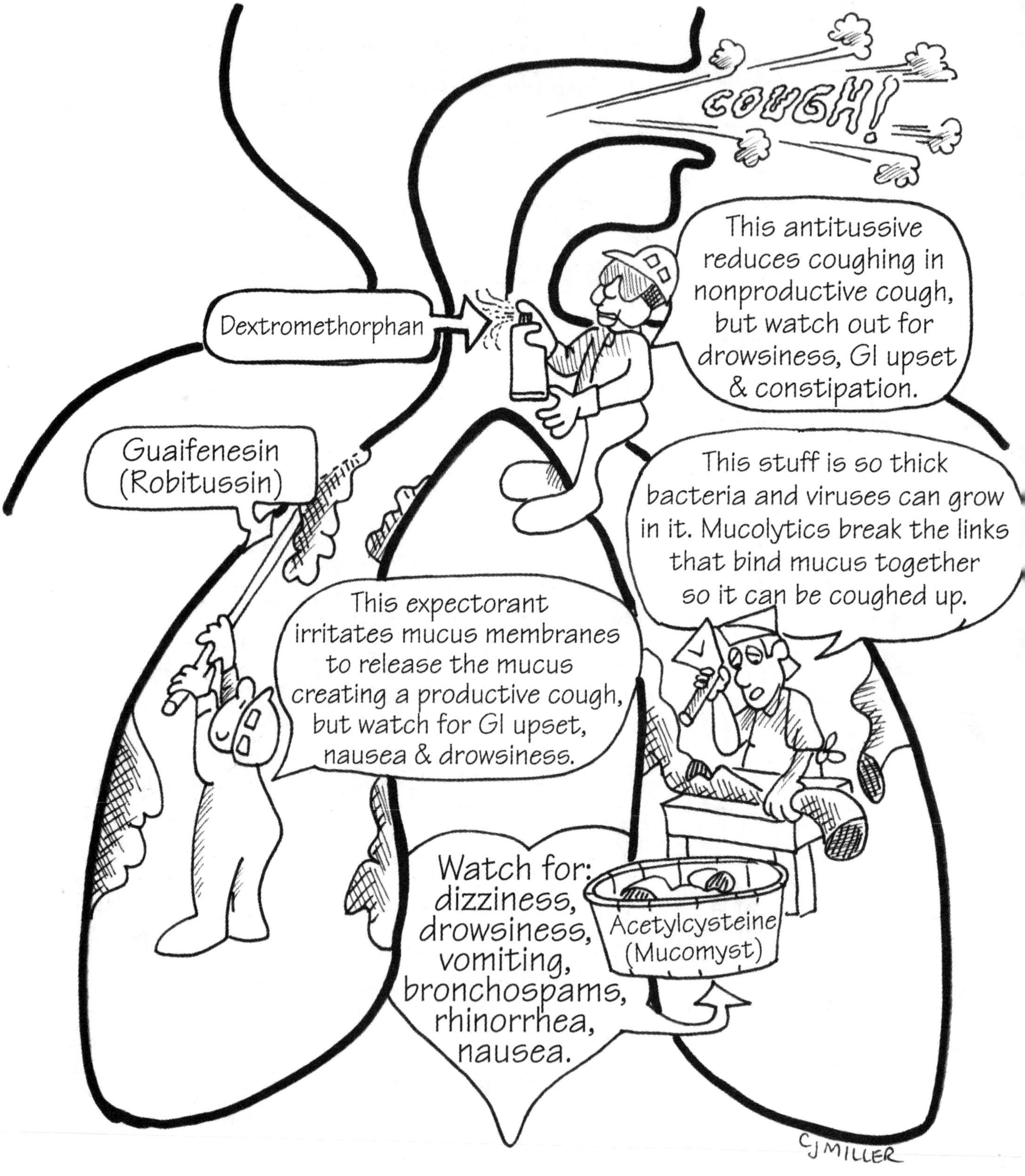

COUGH!
Dextromethorphan
This antitussive reduces coughing in nonproductive cough, but watch out for drowsiness, GI upset & constipation.
Guaifenesin (Robitussin)
This stuff is so thick bacteria and viruses can grow in it. Mucolytics break the links that bind mucus together so it can be coughed up.
This expectorant irritates mucus membranes to release the mucus creating a productive cough, but watch for GI upset, nausea & drowsiness.
Watch for: dizziness, drowsiness, vomiting, bronchospams, rhinorrhea, nausea.
Acetylcysteine (Mucomyst)
CJ MILLER

Bronchodilators

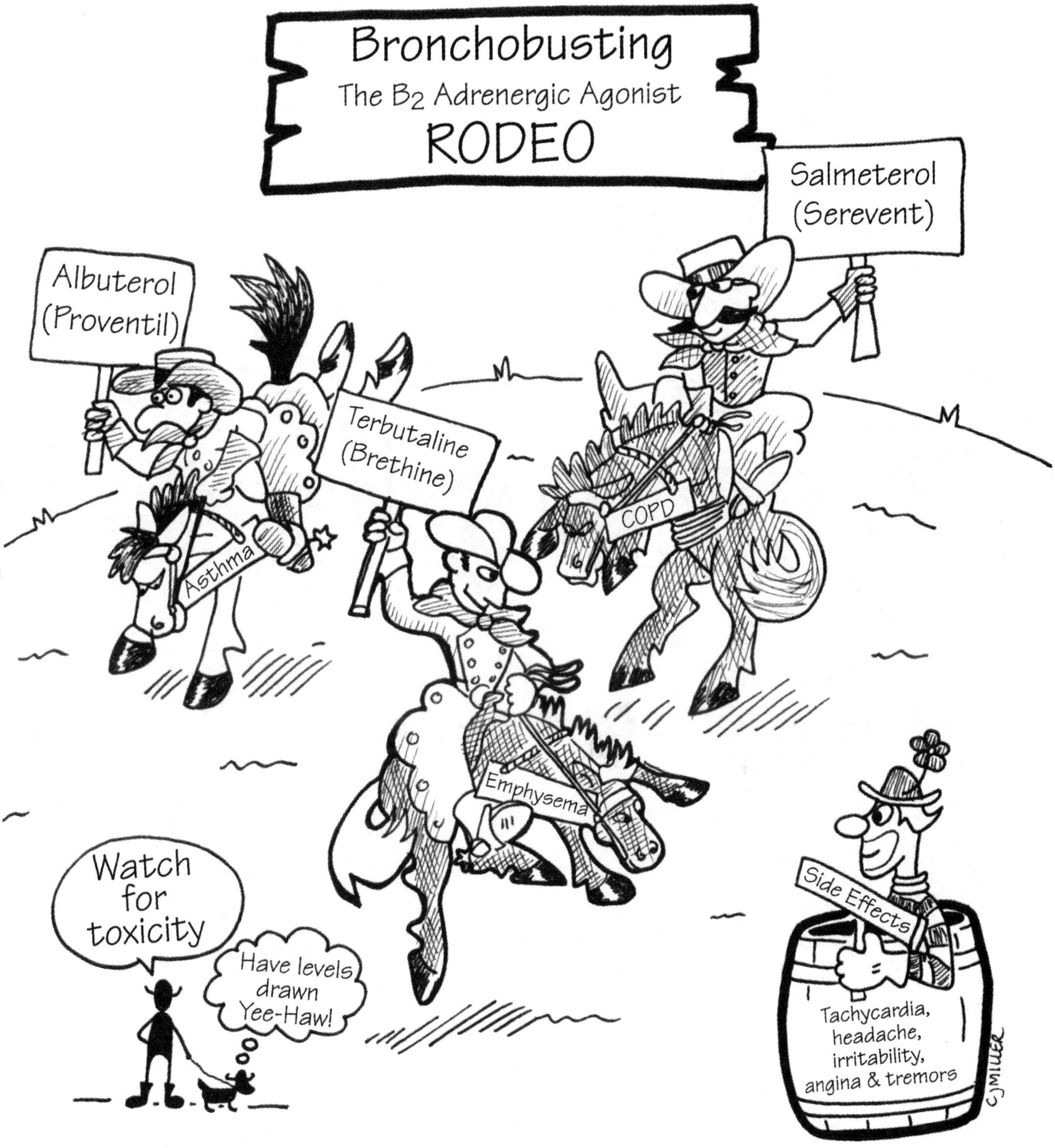

Cetirizine (Zyrtec)

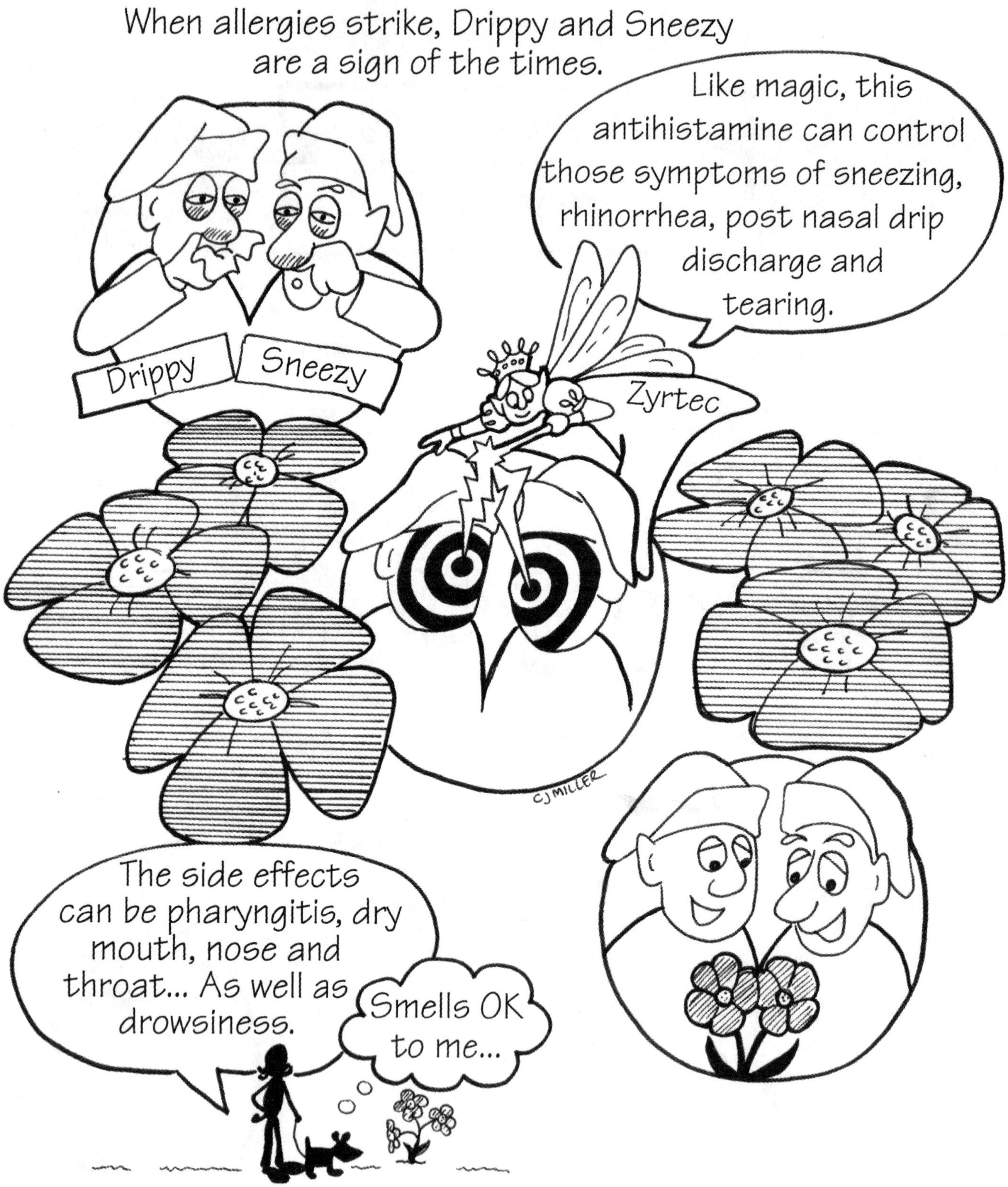
When allergies strike, Drippy and Sneezy are a sign of the times.
Like magic, this antihistamine can control those symptoms of sneezing, rhinorrhea, post nasal drip discharge and tearing.
Drippy
Sneezy
Zyrtec
CJ MILLER
The side effects can be pharyngitis, dry mouth, nose and throat... As well as drowsiness.
Smells OK to me...

Pulmicort (Budesonide)

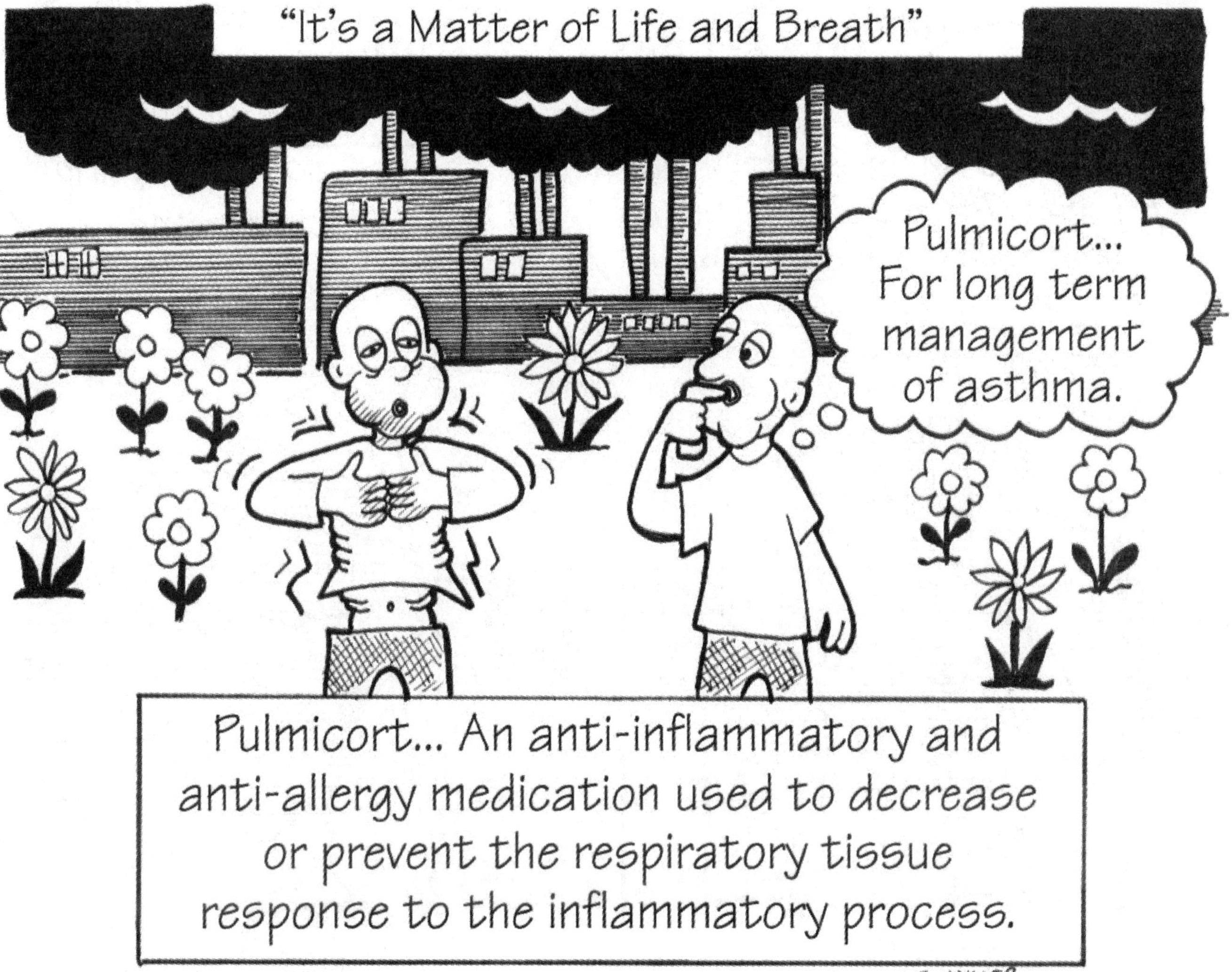
"It's a Matter of Life and Breath"
Pulmicort... For long term management of asthma.
Pulmicort... An anti-inflammatory and anti-allergy medication used to decrease or prevent the respiratory tissue response to the inflammatory process.
CJMILLER

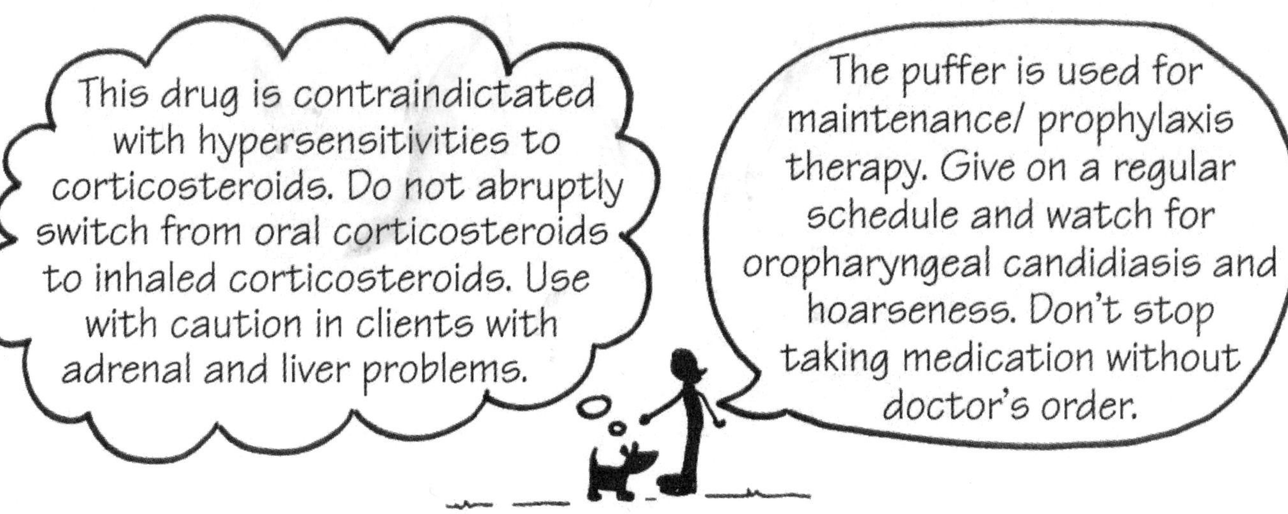
This drug is contraindictated with hypersensitivities to corticosteroids. Do not abruptly switch from oral corticosteroids to inhaled corticosteroids. Use with caution in clients with adrenal and liver problems.
The puffer is used for maintenance/ prophylaxis therapy. Give on a regular schedule and watch for oropharyngeal candidiasis and hoarseness. Don't stop taking medication without doctor's order.

Aluminum Hydroxide (Amphojel)

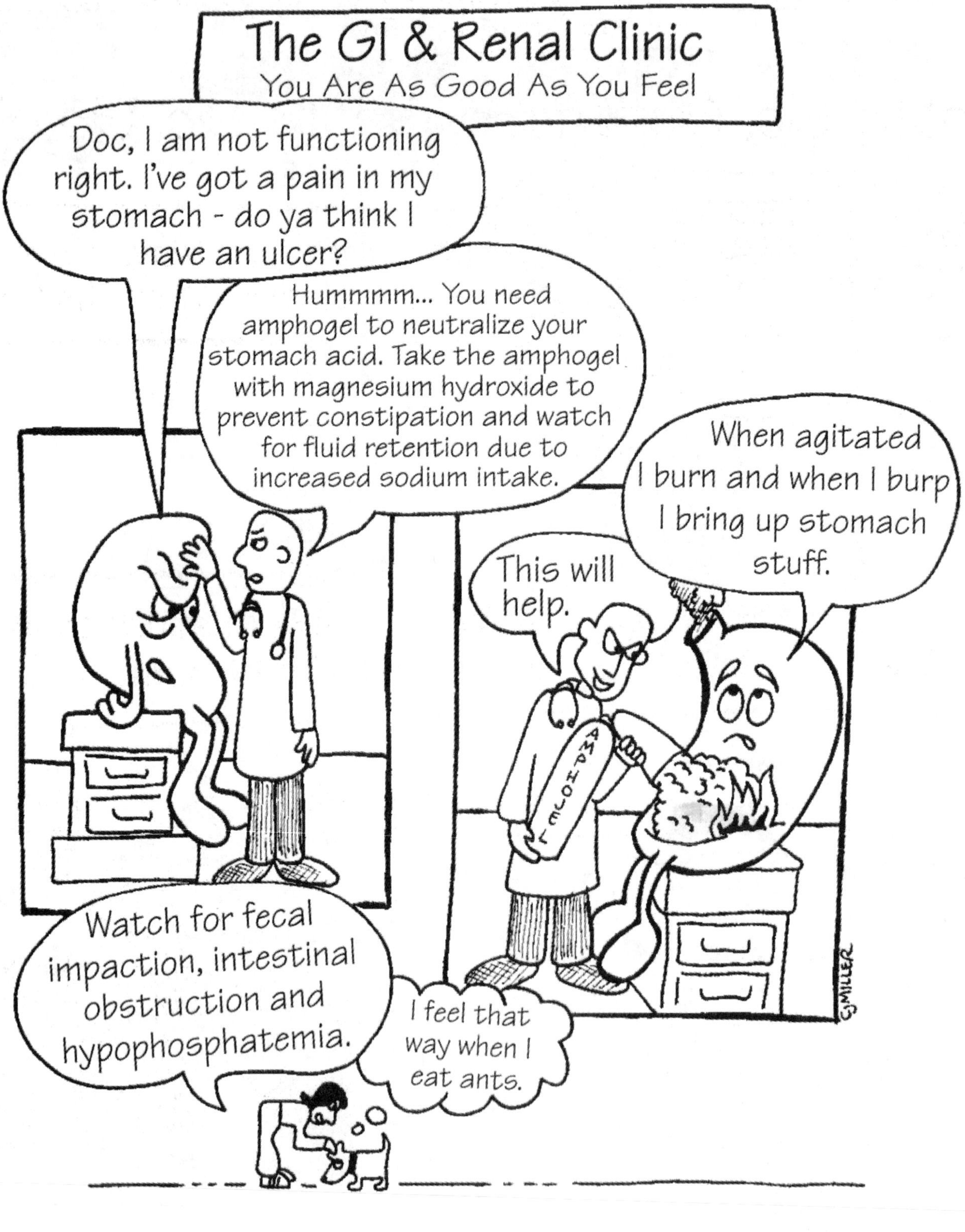
The GI & Renal Clinic
You Are As Good As You Feel
Doc, I am not functioning right. I've got a pain in my stomach - do ya think I have an ulcer?
Hummmm... You need amphogel to neutralize your stomach acid. Take the amphogel with magnesium hydroxide to prevent constipation and watch for fluid retention due to increased sodium intake.
This will help.
When agitated I burn and when I burp I bring up stomach stuff.
AMPHOJEL
CJ MILLER
Watch for fecal impaction, intestinal obstruction and hypophosphatemia.
I feel that way when I eat ants.

Antidiarrheals

Loperamide (Imodium) and Diphenoxylate Hydrochloride (Lomotil)
- With Atropine Sulfate -

Gotta Go, Gotta Go, Gotta Go, Go Go!

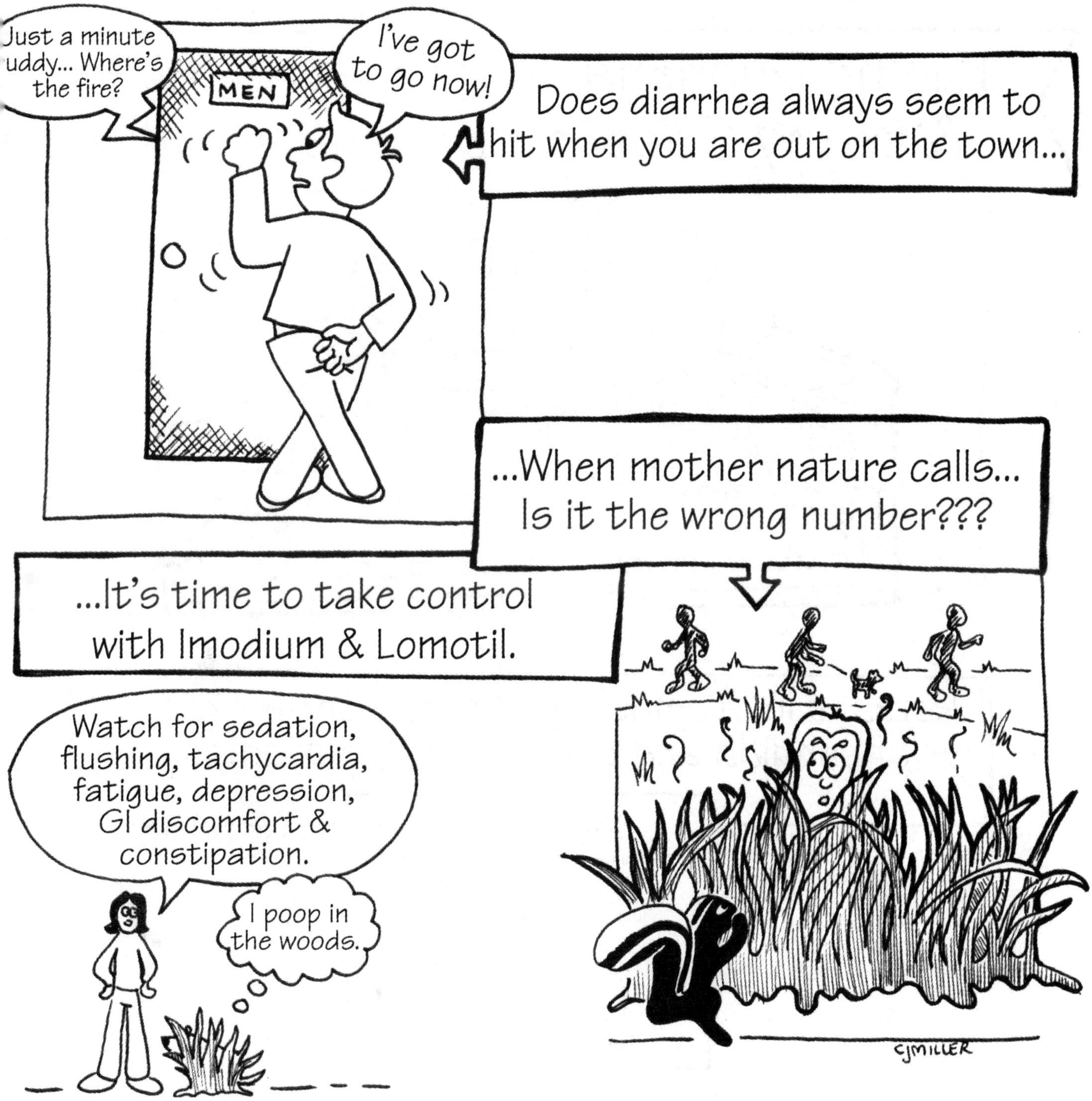

Just a minute uddy... Where's the fire?
MEN
I've got to go now!
Does diarrhea always seem to hit when you are out on the town...
...When mother nature calls... Is it the wrong number???
...It's time to take control with Imodium & Lomotil.
Watch for sedation, flushing, tachycardia, fatigue, depression, GI discomfort & constipation.
I poop in the woods.
CJMILLER

H_2 Blockers

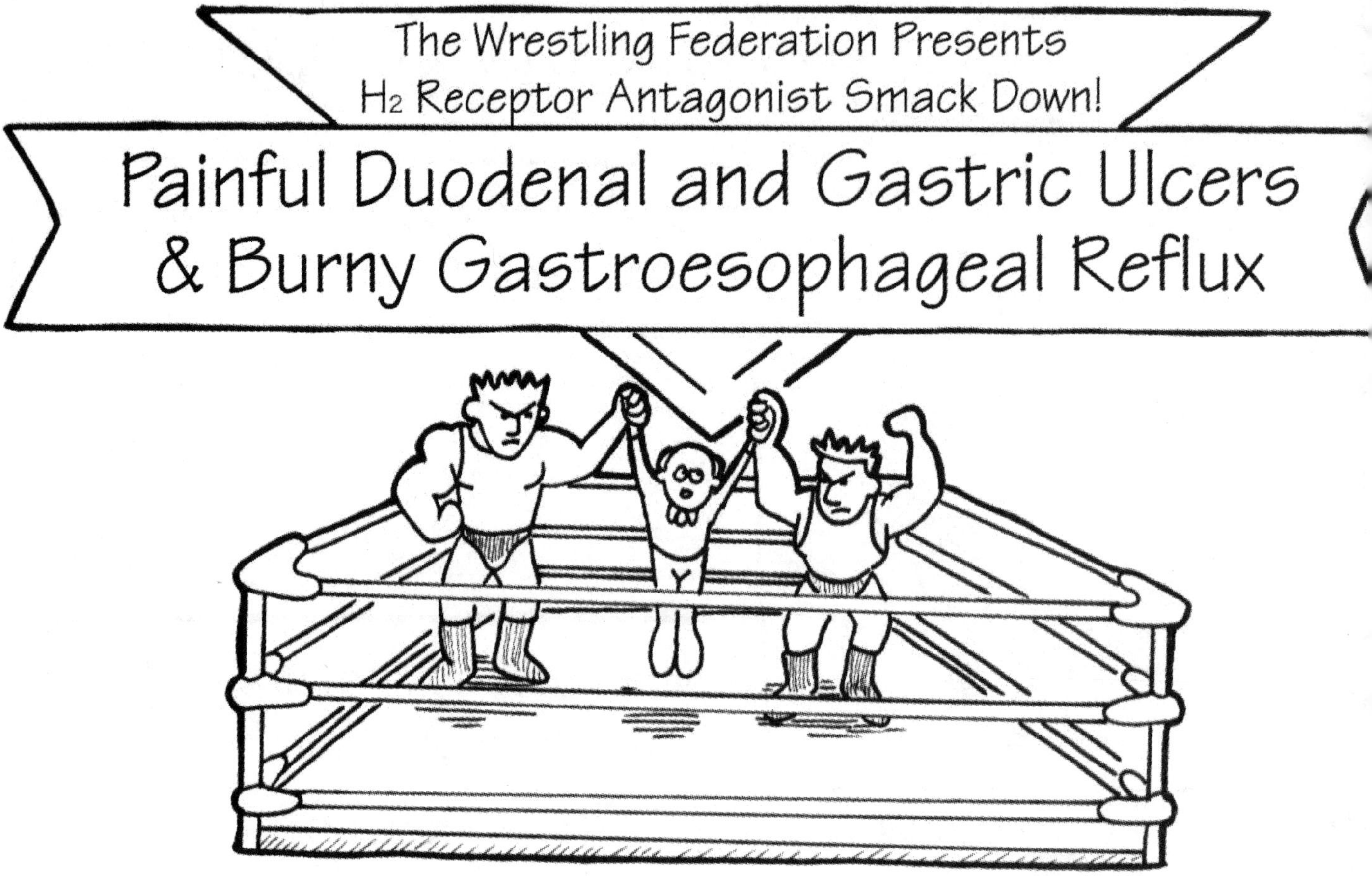
The Wrestling Federation Presents
H_2 Receptor Antagonist Smack Down!
Painful Duodenal and Gastric Ulcers
& Burny Gastroesophageal Reflux

Decrease in stomach acid may increase growth of candida and bacteria in the stomach

Watch for pneumonia due to colonization and increased pH in stomach.

CJMILLER

Kayexalate

(Sodium Polystyrene Sulfonate)

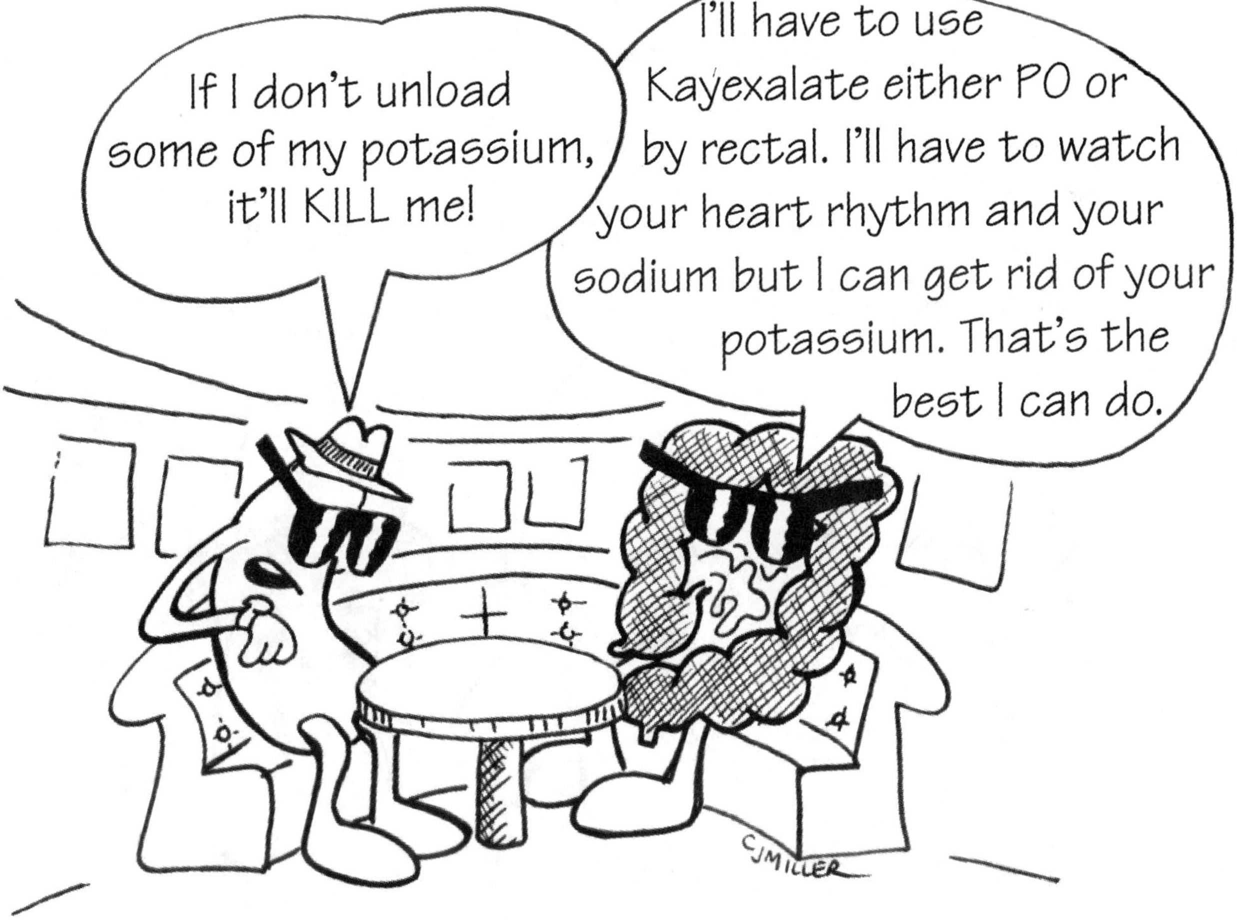
If I don't unload some of my potassium, it'll KILL me!
I'll have to use Kayexalate either PO or by rectal. I'll have to watch your heart rhythm and your sodium but I can get rid of your potassium. That's the best I can do.
CJMILLER

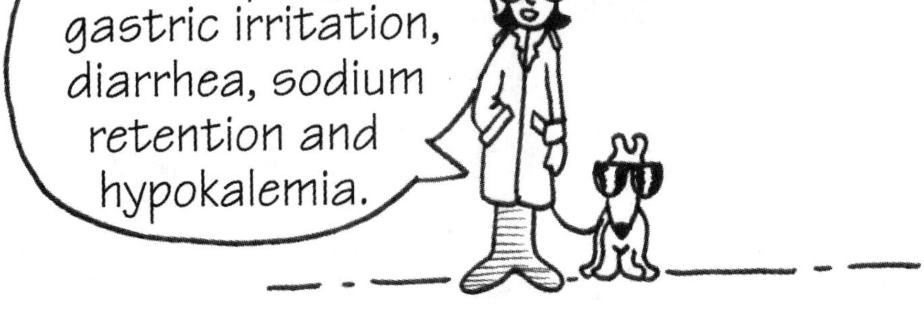
Watch for constipation, gastric irritation, diarrhea, sodium retention and hypokalemia.

Lactulose

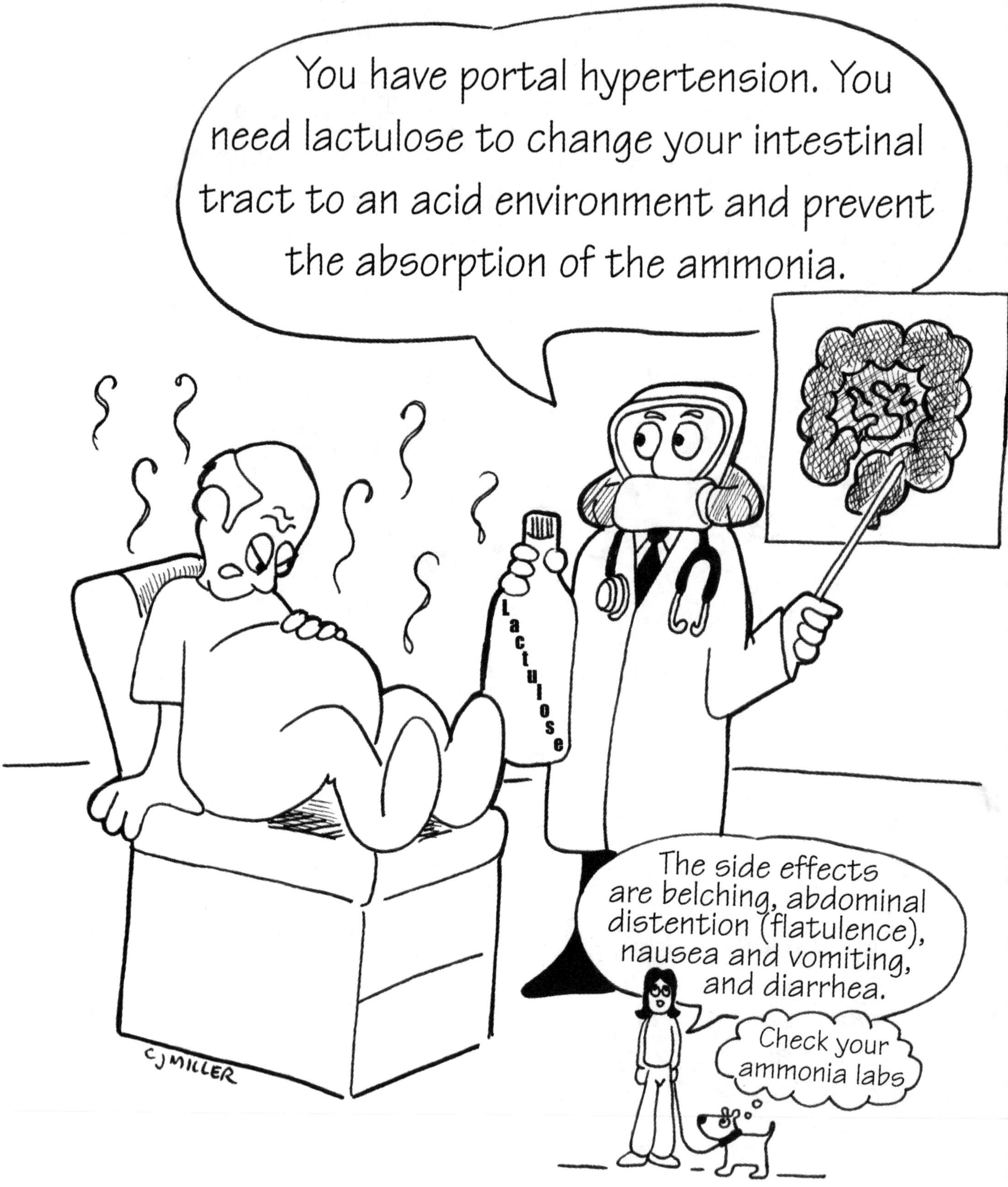
You have portal hypertension. You need lactulose to change your intestinal tract to an acid environment and prevent the absorption of the ammonia.
Lactulose
The side effects are belching, abdominal distention (flatulence), nausea and vomiting, and diarrhea.
Check your ammonia labs
CJ MILLER

Magnesium Hydroxide (Milk of Magnesia)

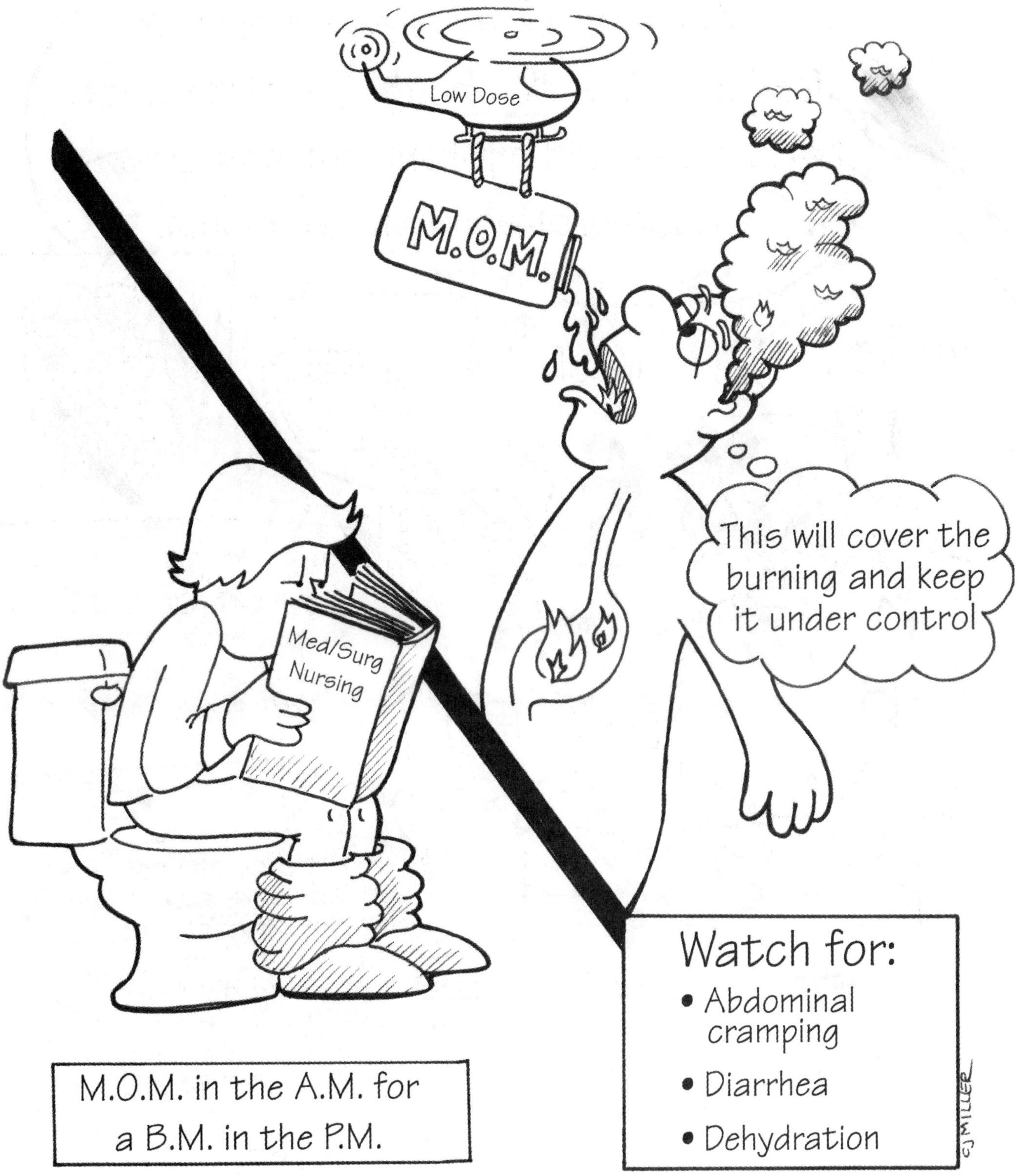
Low Dose
M.O.M.
This will cover the burning and keep it under control
Med/Surg Nursing
M.O.M. in the A.M. for a B.M. in the P.M.
Watch for:
• Abdominal cramping
• Diarrhea
• Dehydration
CJ MILLER

Metoclopramide (Reglan)

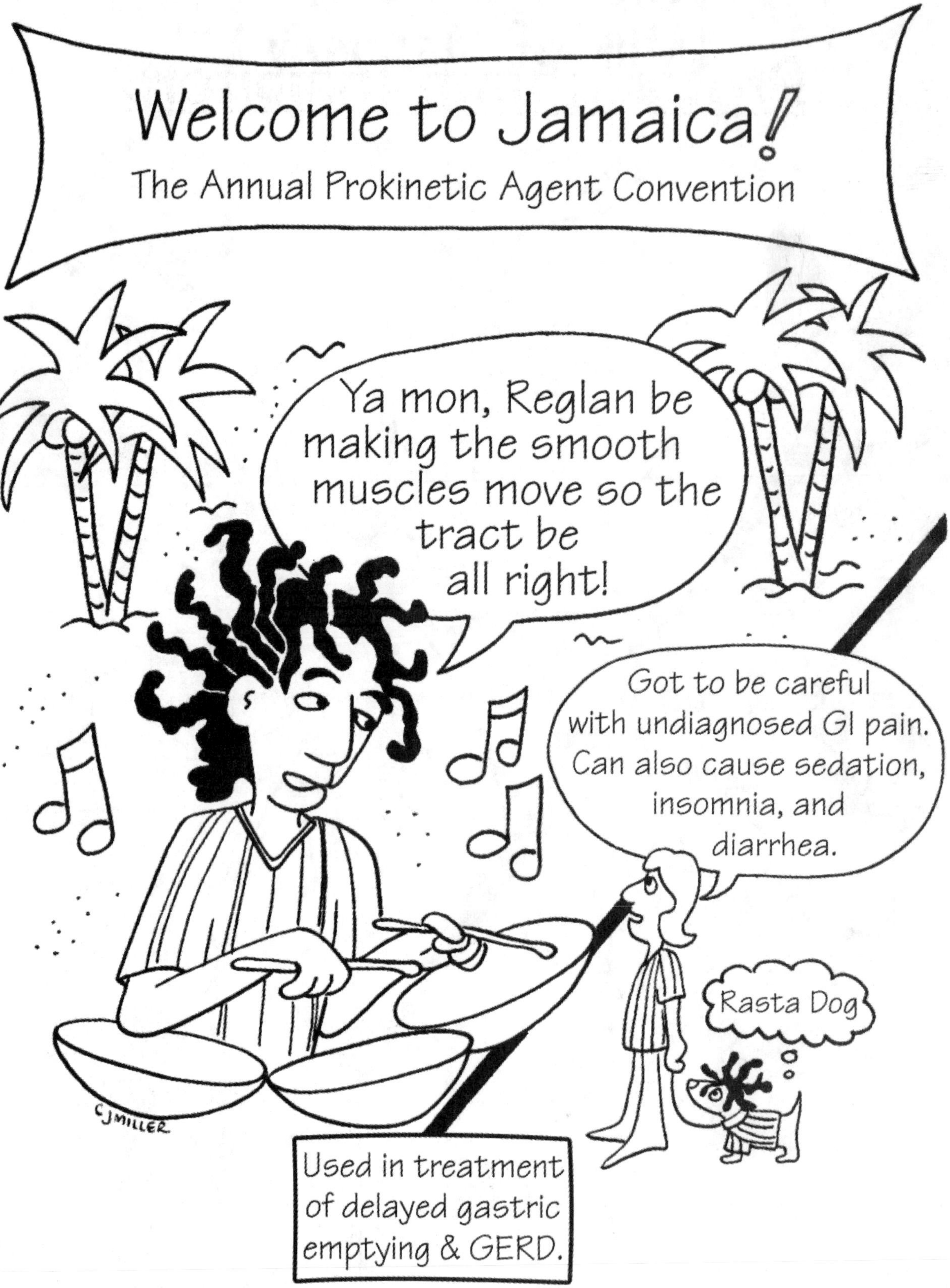
Welcome to Jamaica!
The Annual Prokinetic Agent Convention
Ya mon, Reglan be making the smooth muscles move so the tract be all right!
Got to be careful with undiagnosed GI pain. Can also cause sedation, insomnia, and diarrhea.
Rasta Dog
Used in treatment of delayed gastric emptying & GERD.
CJMILLER

Proton Pump Inhibitors

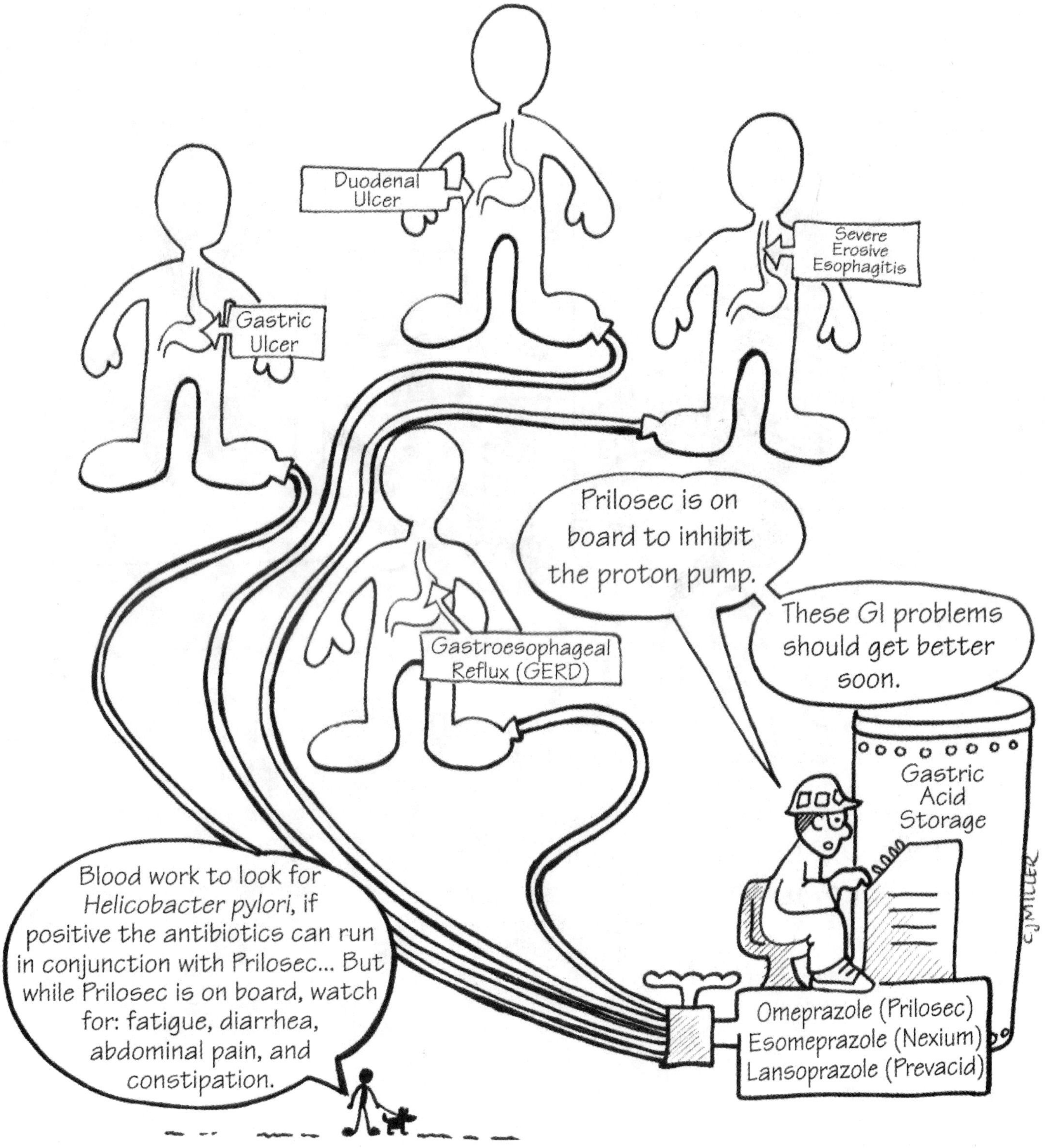

Duodenal Ulcer
Severe Erosive Esophagitis
Gastric Ulcer
Prilosec is on board to inhibit the proton pump.
These GI problems should get better soon.
Gastroesophageal Reflux (GERD)
Gastric Acid Storage
CJ MILLER
Blood work to look for *Helicobacter pylori*, if positive the antibiotics can run in conjunction with Prilosec... But while Prilosec is on board, watch for: fatigue, diarrhea, abdominal pain, and constipation.
Omeprazole (Prilosec)
Esomeprazole (Nexium)
Lansoprazole (Prevacid)

Prochlorperazine (Compazine)

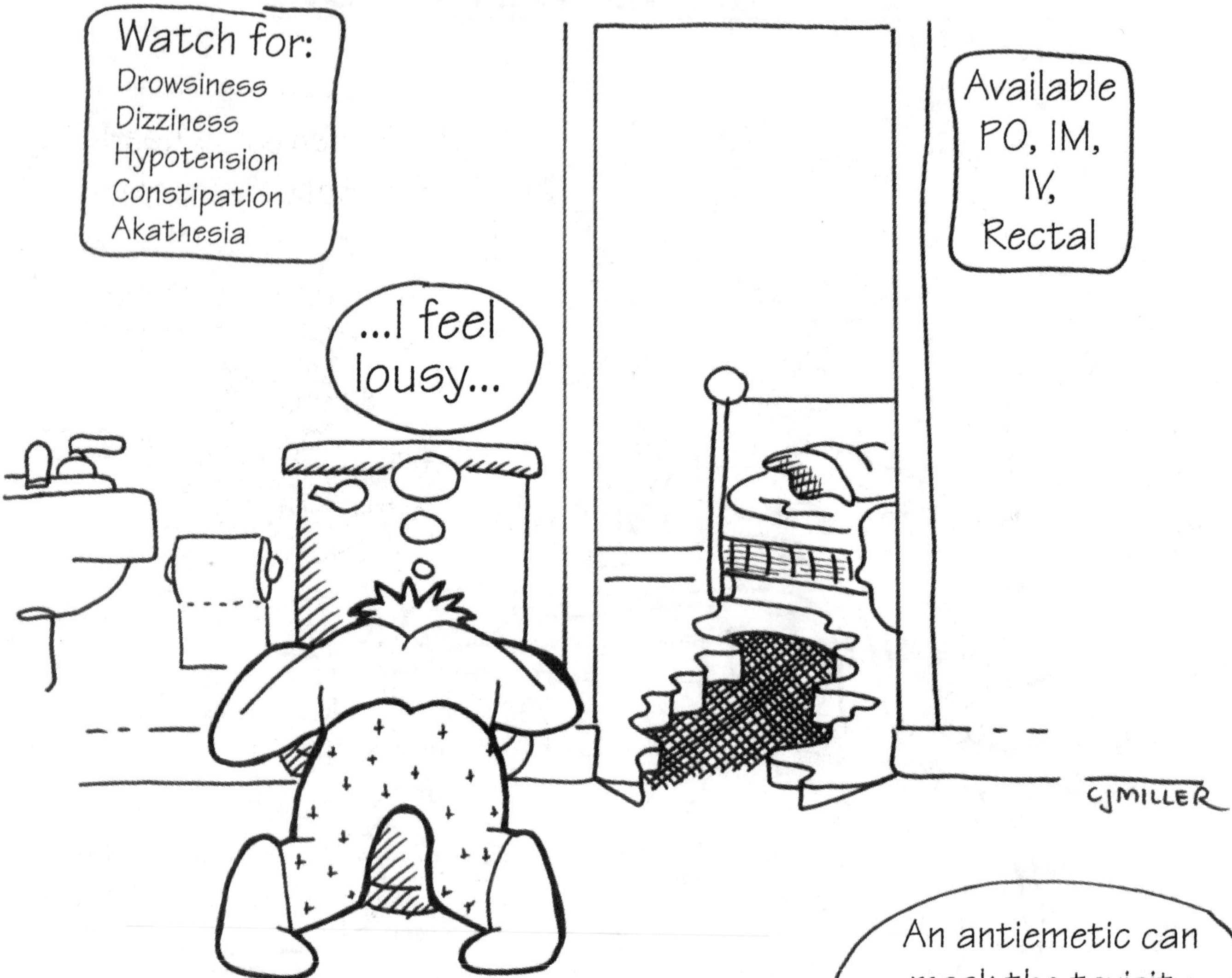
Watch for:
Drowsiness
Dizziness
Hypotension
Constipation
Akathesia
Available PO, IM, IV, Rectal
...I feel lousy...
CJMILLER

When you are in a rut and can't stop hugging the bowl, it's time for Compazine, an antiemetic for severe nausea and vomiting.

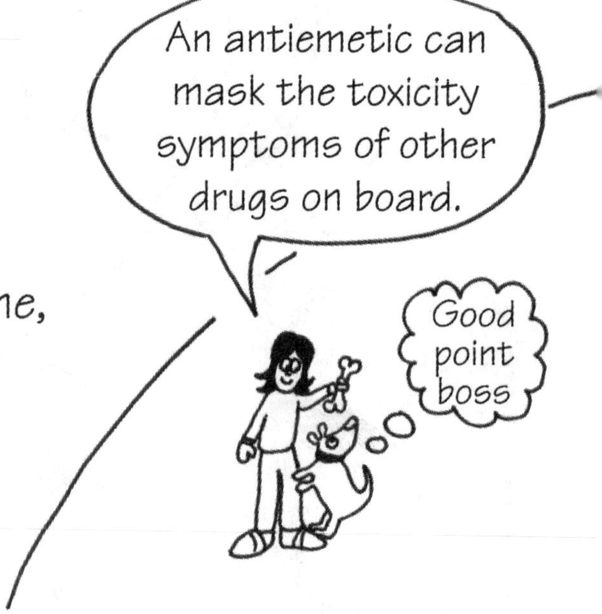
An antiemetic can mask the toxicity symptoms of other drugs on board.
Good point boss

Promethazine (Phenergan)

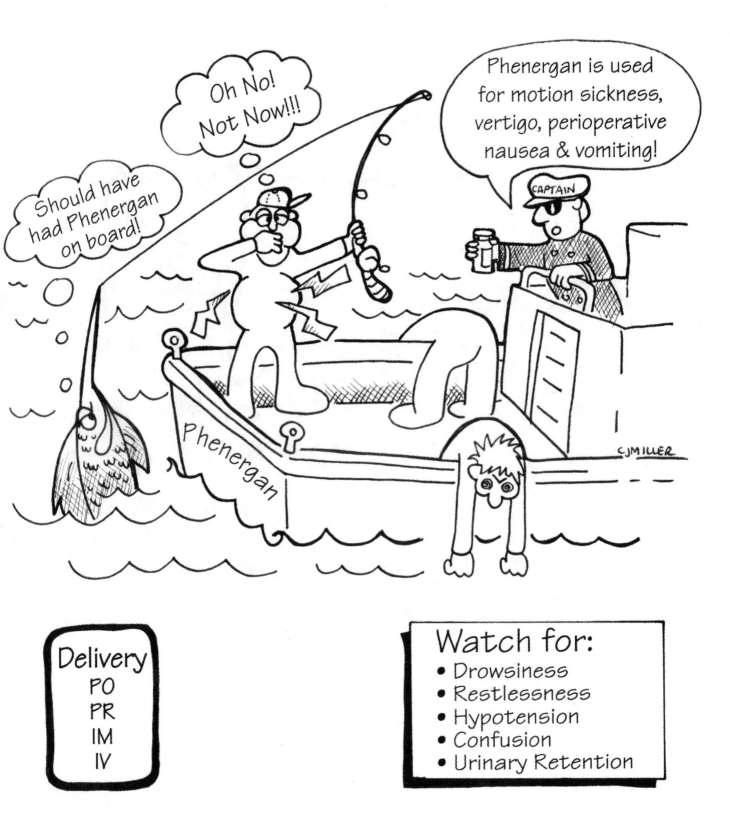

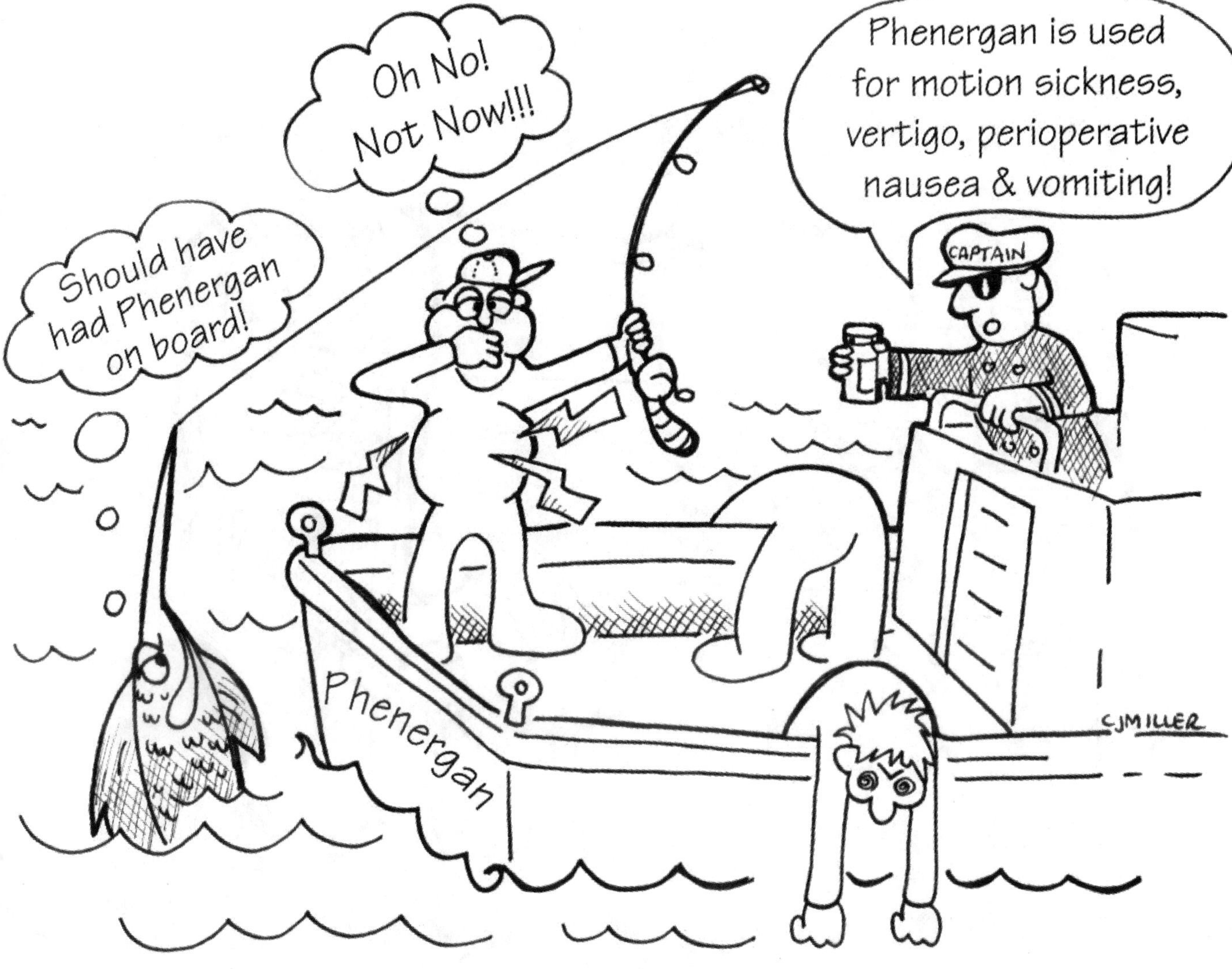
Should have had Phenergan on board!
Oh No! Not Now!!!
Phenergan is used for motion sickness, vertigo, perioperative nausea & vomiting!
CAPTAIN
Phenergan
CJMILLER

Delivery
PO
PR
IM
IV

Watch for:
- Drowsiness
- Restlessness
- Hypotension
- Confusion
- Urinary Retention

Psyllium (Metamucil)

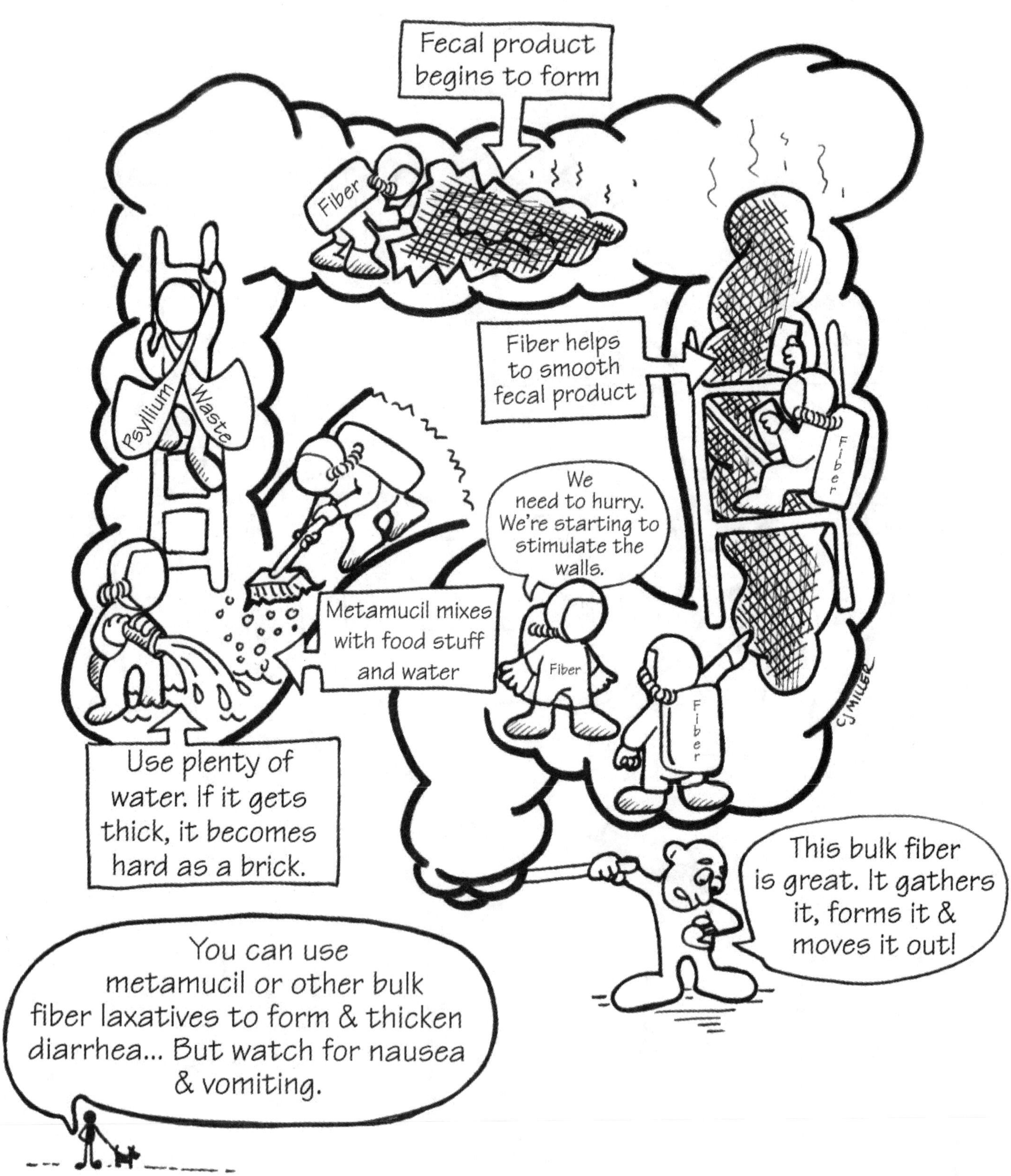

Fecal product begins to form
Fiber
Psyllium
Waste
Fiber helps to smooth fecal product
Fiber
We need to hurry. We're starting to stimulate the walls.
Metamucil mixes with food stuff and water
Fiber
Fiber
CJ MILLER
Use plenty of water. If it gets thick, it becomes hard as a brick.
This bulk fiber is great. It gathers it, forms it & moves it out!
You can use metamucil or other bulk fiber laxatives to form & thicken diarrhea... But watch for nausea & vomiting.

Bumetanide (Bumex)

"Gets the Fluid on the Move"

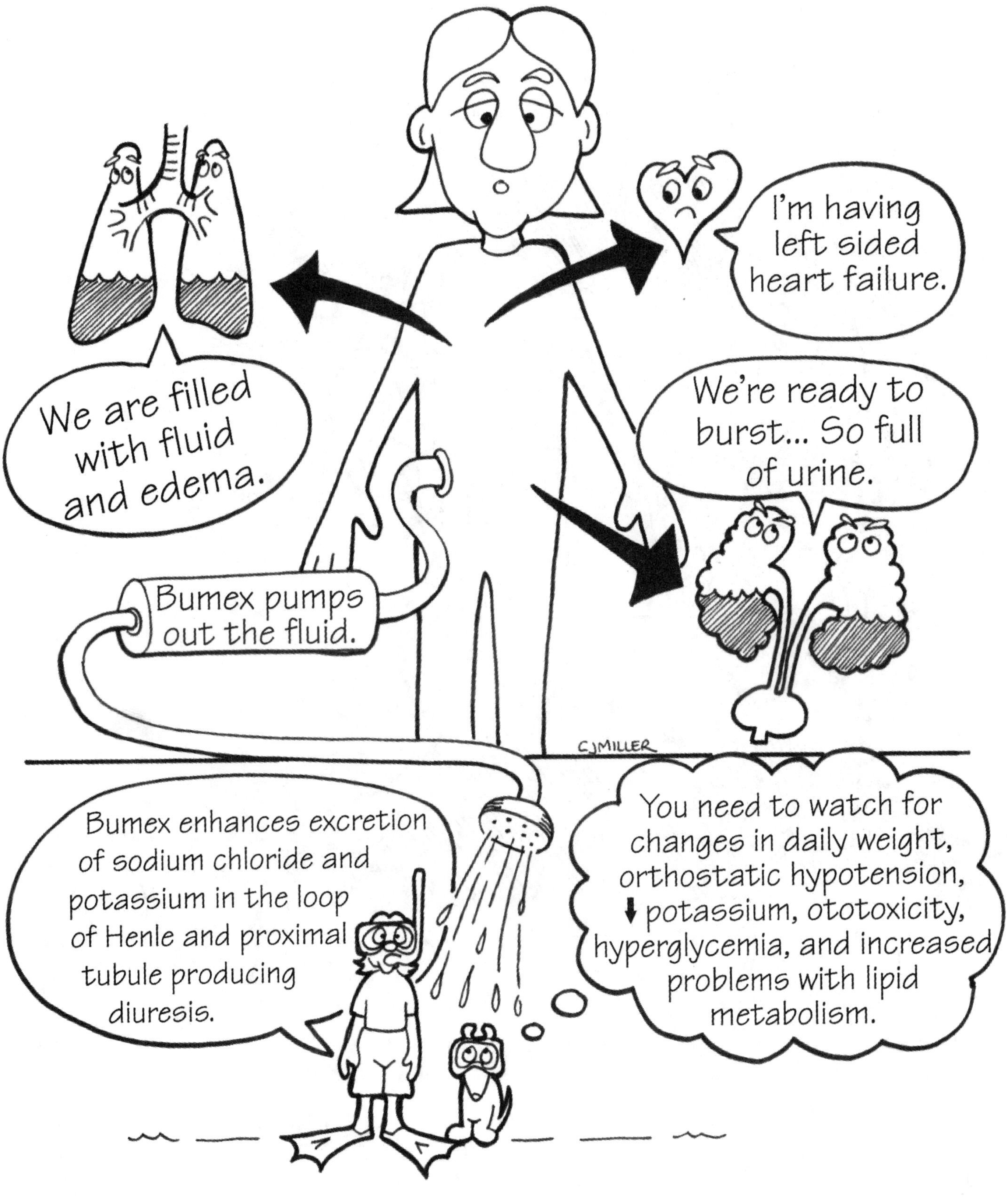

I'm having left sided heart failure.
We are filled with fluid and edema.
We're ready to burst... So full of urine.
Bumex pumps out the fluid.
CJMILLER
Bumex enhances excretion of sodium chloride and potassium in the loop of Henle and proximal tubule producing diuresis.
You need to watch for changes in daily weight, orthostatic hypotension, ↓ potassium, ototoxicity, hyperglycemia, and increased problems with lipid metabolism.

Diuretic Water Slide

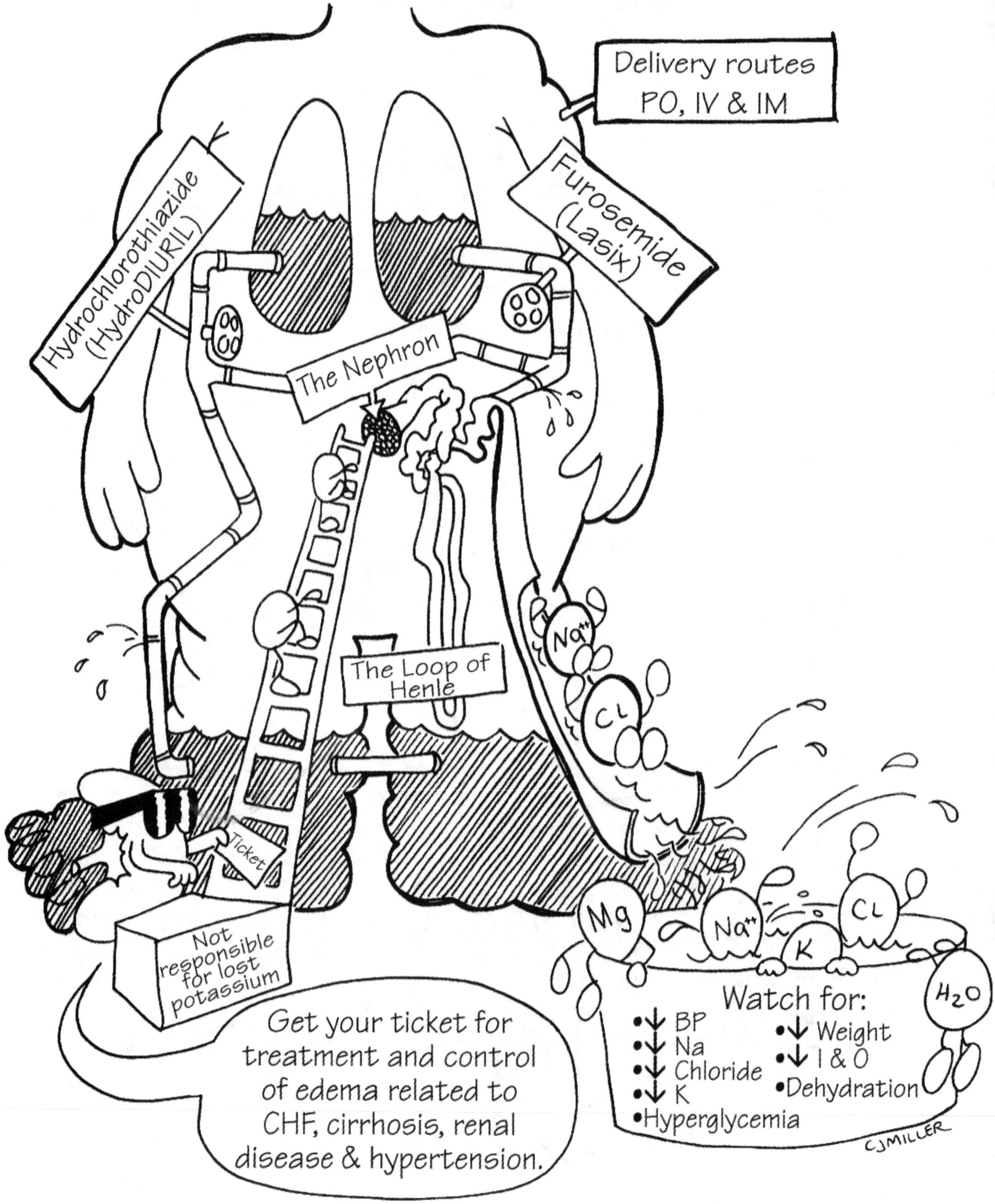

Osmitrol (Mannitol)

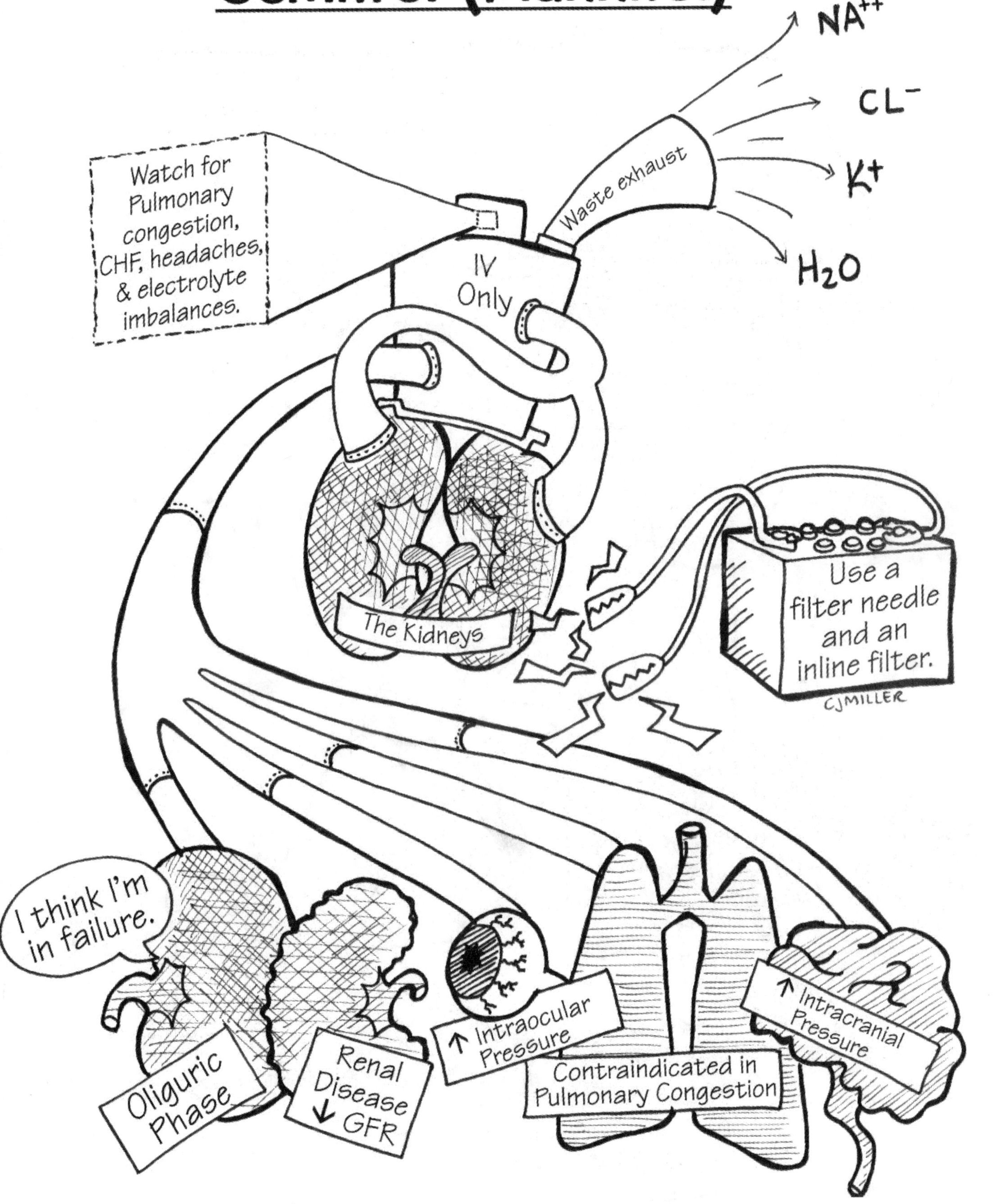

Spironolactone (Aldactone)

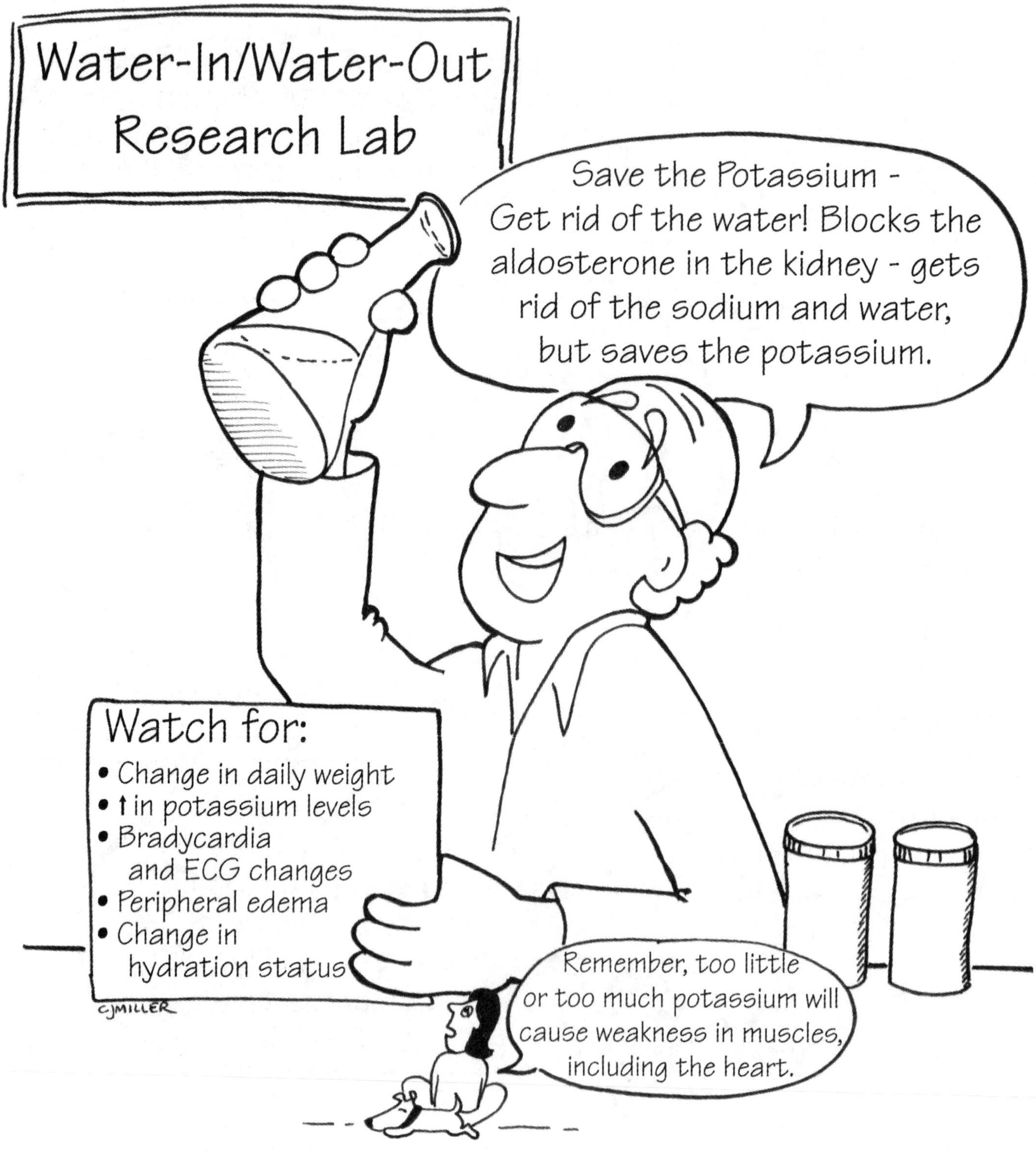
Water-In/Water-Out
Research Lab
Save the Potassium - Get rid of the water! Blocks the aldosterone in the kidney - gets rid of the sodium and water, but saves the potassium.
Watch for:
• Change in daily weight
• ↑ in potassium levels
• Bradycardia and ECG changes
• Peripheral edema
• Change in hydration status
CJMILLER
Remember, too little or too much potassium will cause weakness in muscles, including the heart.

Bupropion (Wellbutrin and Zyban)

"Getting Well with Wellbutrin."

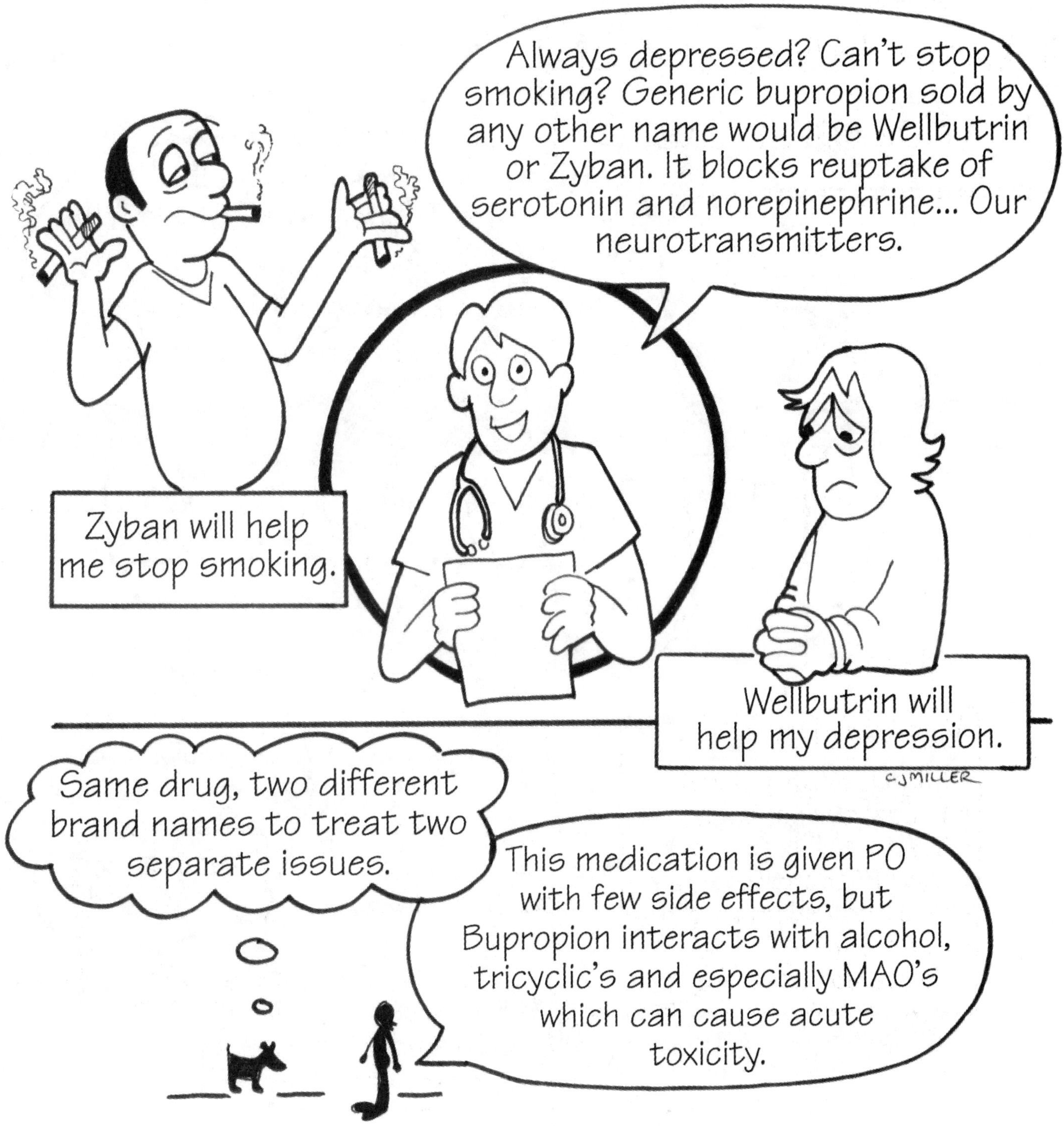
Always depressed? Can't stop smoking? Generic bupropion sold by any other name would be Wellbutrin or Zyban. It blocks reuptake of serotonin and norepinephrine... Our neurotransmitters.
Zyban will help me stop smoking.
Wellbutrin will help my depression.
CJMILLER
Same drug, two different brand names to treat two separate issues.
This medication is given PO with few side effects, but Bupropion interacts with alcohol, tricyclic's and especially MAO's which can cause acute toxicity.

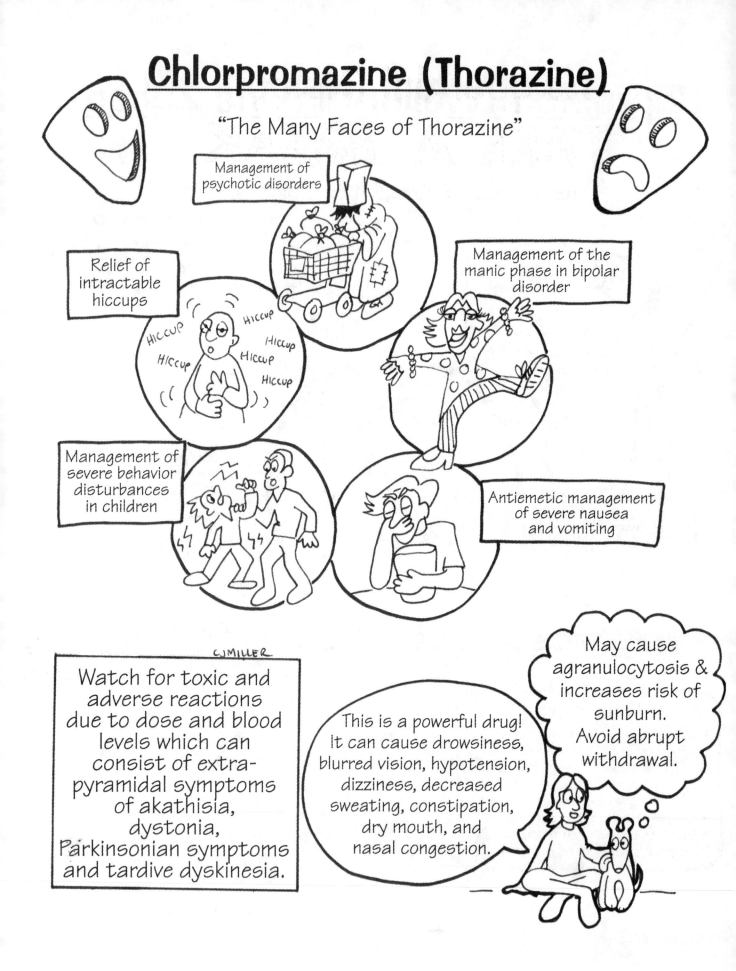

Chlorpromazine (Thorazine)

"The Many Faces of Thorazine"

Management of psychotic disorders
Relief of intractable hiccups
HICCUP
HICCUP
Hiccup
HICCUP
HICCUP
HICCUP
Management of the manic phase in bipolar disorder
Management of severe behavior disturbances in children
Antiemetic management of severe nausea and vomiting
CJMILLER

Watch for toxic and adverse reactions due to dose and blood levels which can consist of extra-pyramidal symptoms of akathisia, dystonia, Parkinsonian symptoms and tardive dyskinesia.

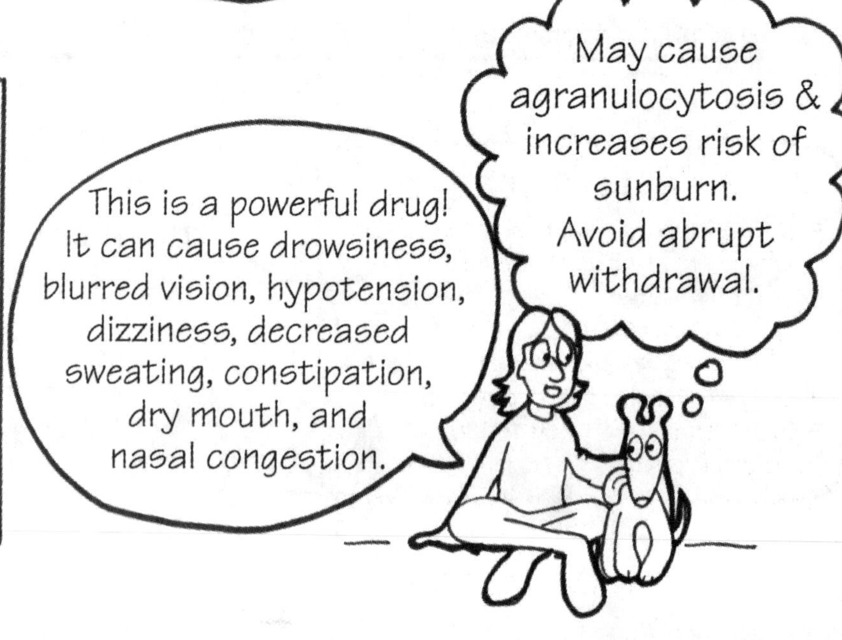
This is a powerful drug! It can cause drowsiness, blurred vision, hypotension, dizziness, decreased sweating, constipation, dry mouth, and nasal congestion.
May cause agranulocytosis & increases risk of sunburn. Avoid abrupt withdrawal.

Haloperidol (Haldol)

TAKE A BREAK

- The Journal of Psychiatric Insight -

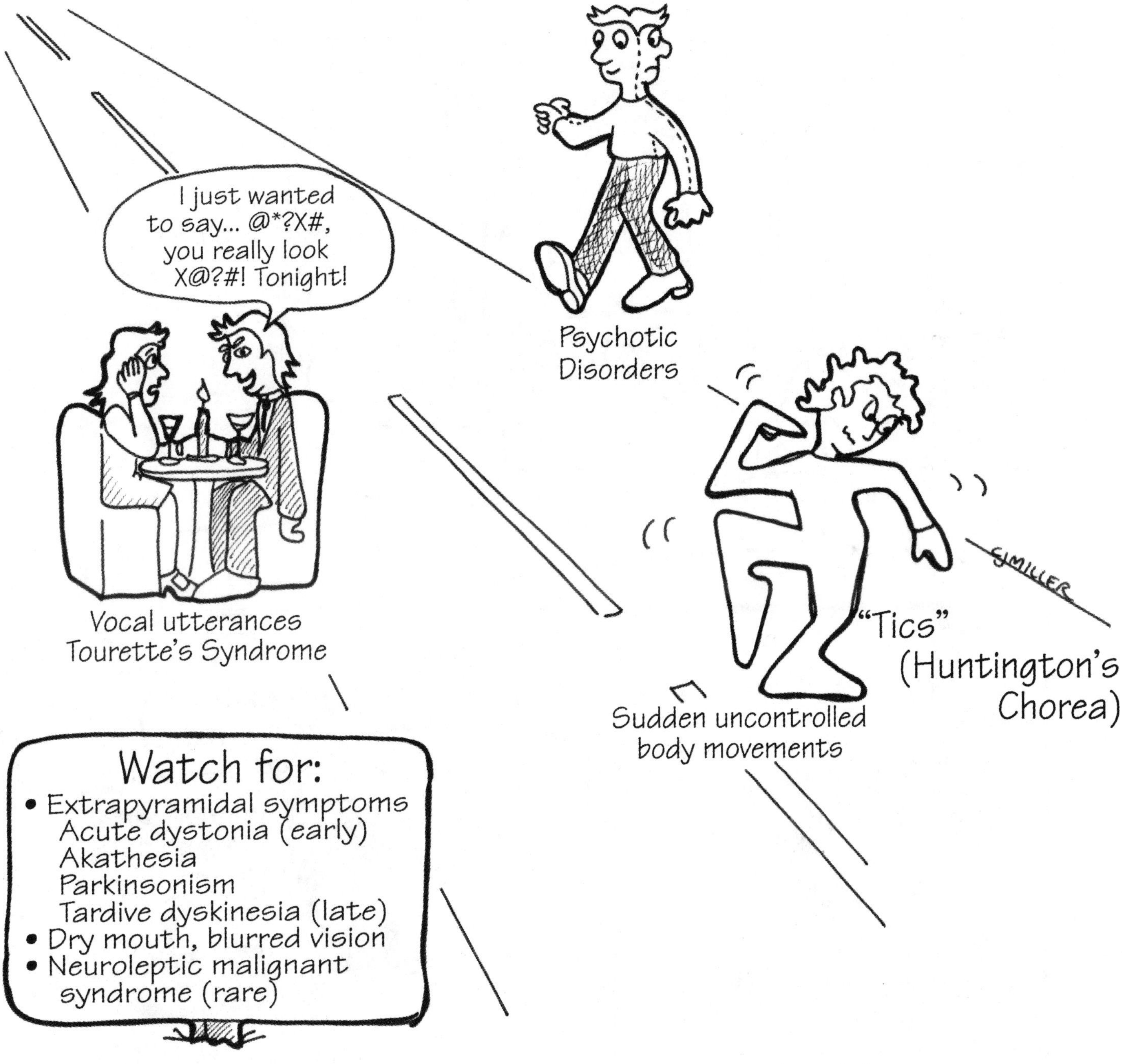

Haldol (Haloperidol) - A new way to get back home.

MAO Inhibitors

Nardil, Marplan & Parnate

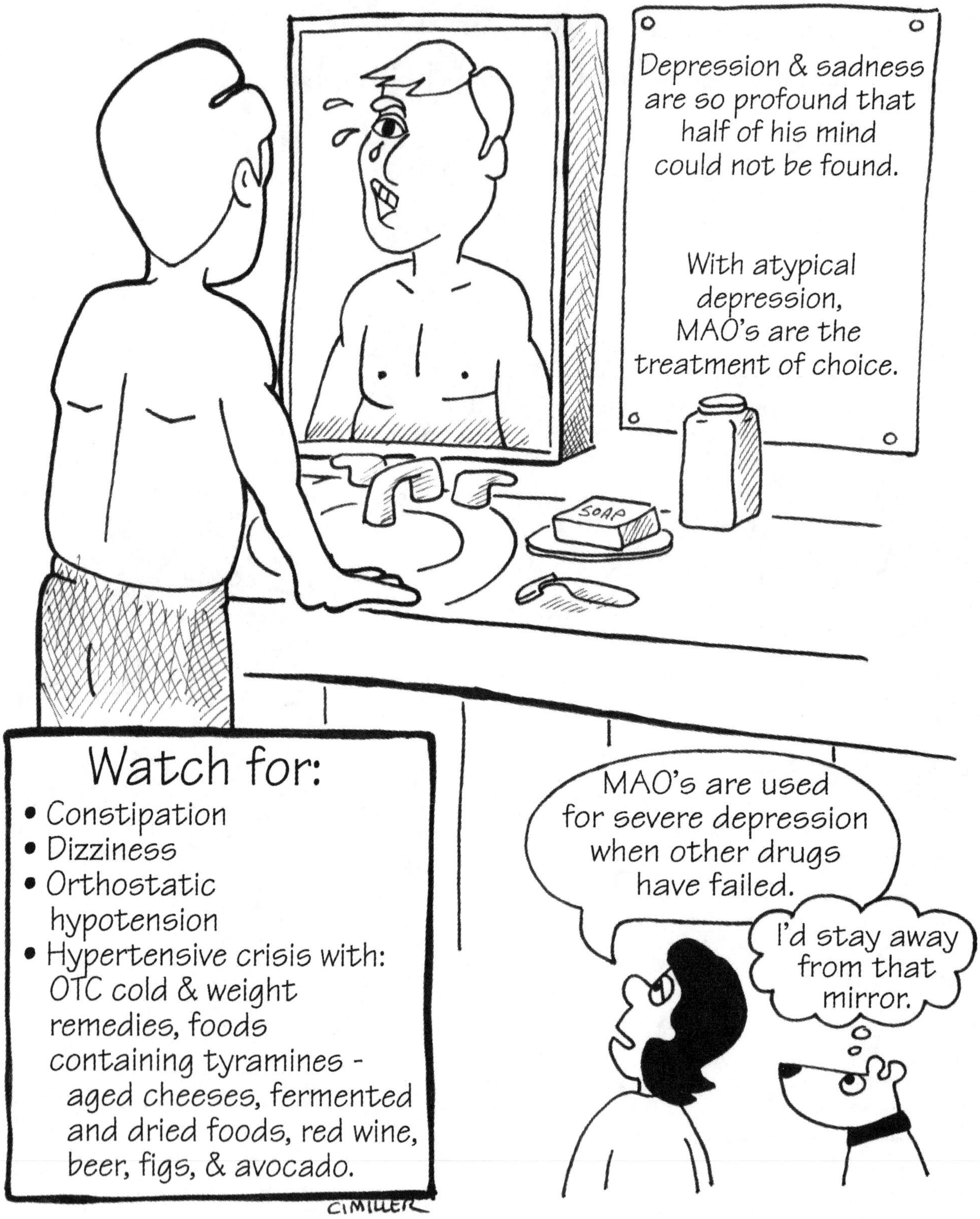
Depression & sadness are so profound that half of his mind could not be found.
With atypical depression, MAO's are the treatment of choice.
SOAP
Watch for:
• Constipation
• Dizziness
• Orthostatic hypotension
• Hypertensive crisis with: OTC cold & weight remedies, foods containing tyramines - aged cheeses, fermented and dried foods, red wine, beer, figs, & avocado.
MAO's are used for severe depression when other drugs have failed.
I'd stay away from that mirror.
C.MILLER

SSRI's

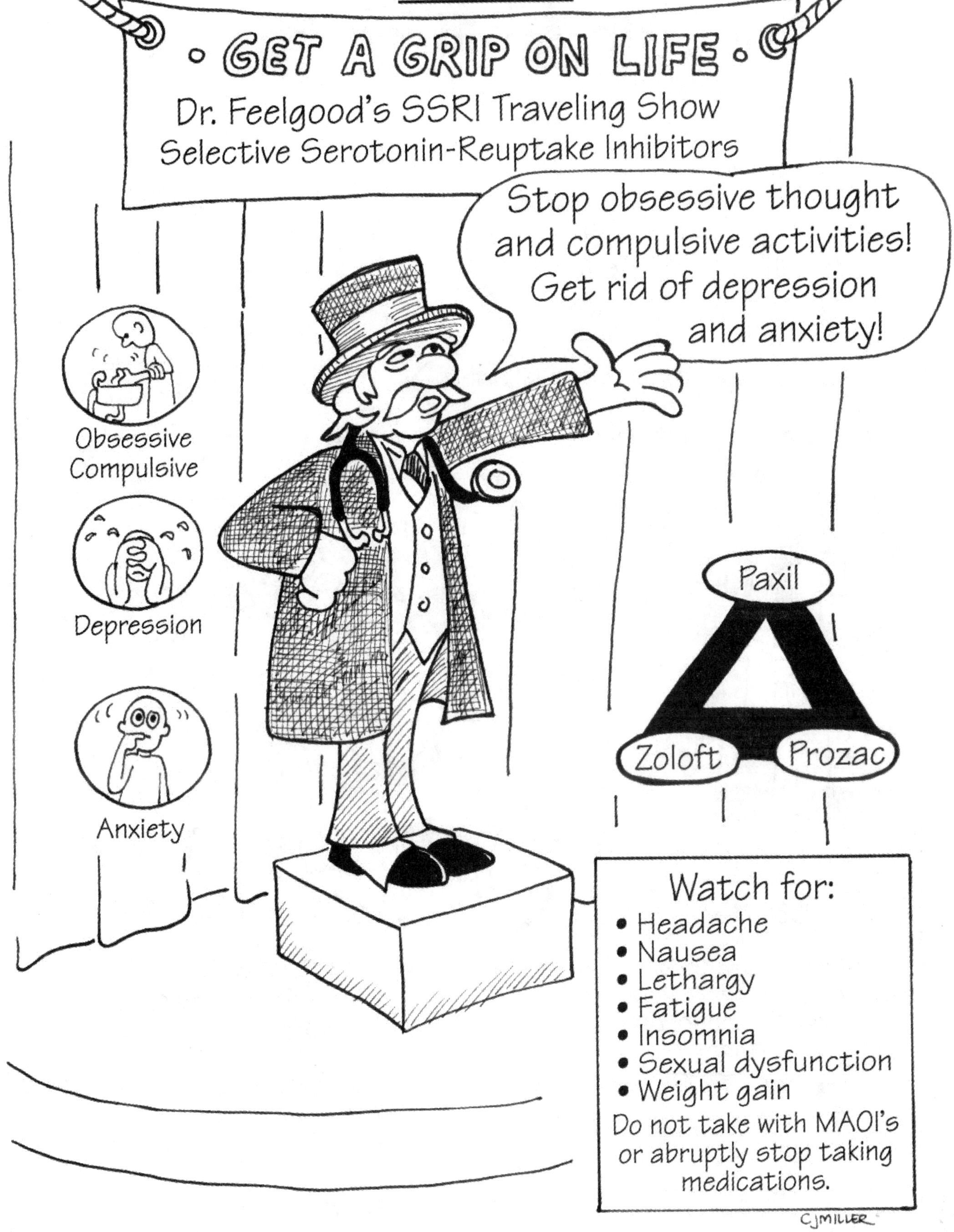

• GET A GRIP ON LIFE •
Dr. Feelgood's SSRI Traveling Show
Selective Serotonin-Reuptake Inhibitors
Stop obsessive thought and compulsive activities! Get rid of depression and anxiety!
Obsessive Compulsive
Depression
Anxiety
Paxil
Zoloft
Prozac
Watch for:
• Headache
• Nausea
• Lethargy
• Fatigue
• Insomnia
• Sexual dysfunction
• Weight gain
Do not take with MAOI's or abruptly stop taking medications.
CJMILLER

Tricyclic Antidepressants

Amitriptyline (Elavil) | Doxepin (Sinequan) | Nortriptyline (Pamelor) | Imipramine (Tofranil)

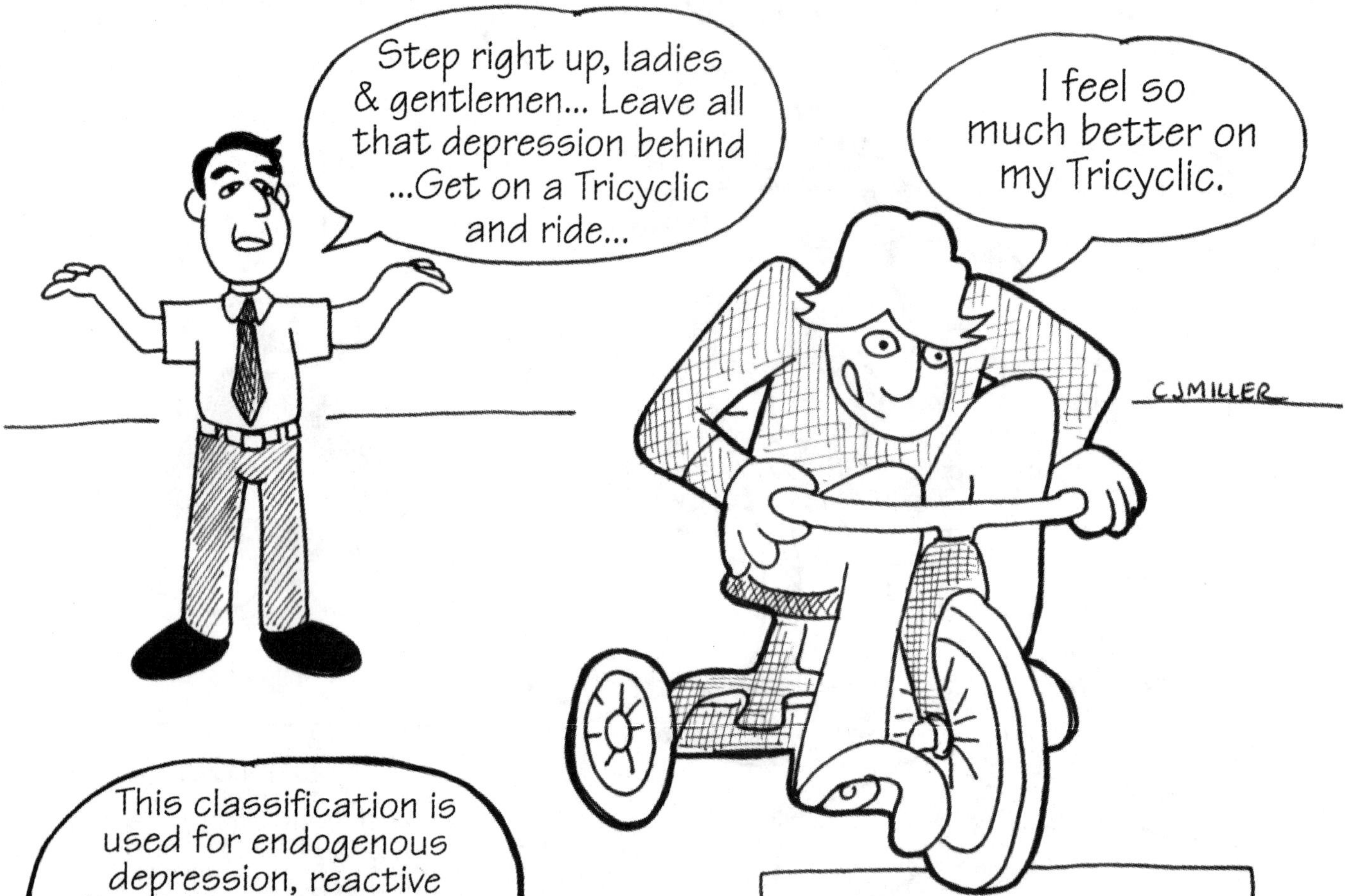

Step right up, ladies & gentlemen... Leave all that depression behind ...Get on a Tricyclic and ride...
I feel so much better on my Tricyclic.
CJMILLER

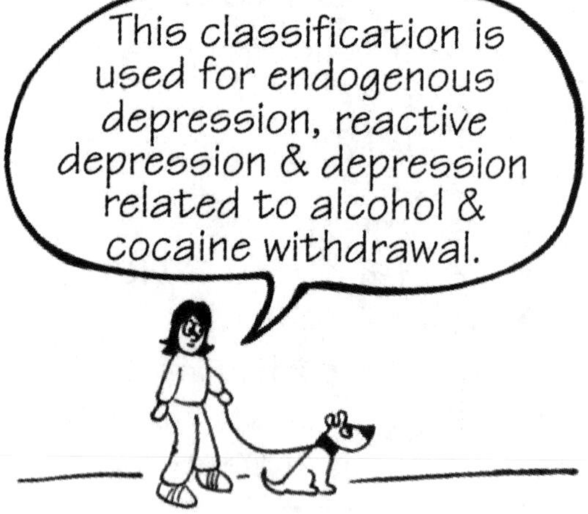

This classification is used for endogenous depression, reactive depression & depression related to alcohol & cocaine withdrawal.

Watch for signs of:
- Sedation
- Orthostatic Hypotension
- Diaphoresis
- Dry Mouth
- Urinary Retention
- Dysrhythmias

Acarbose (Precose)

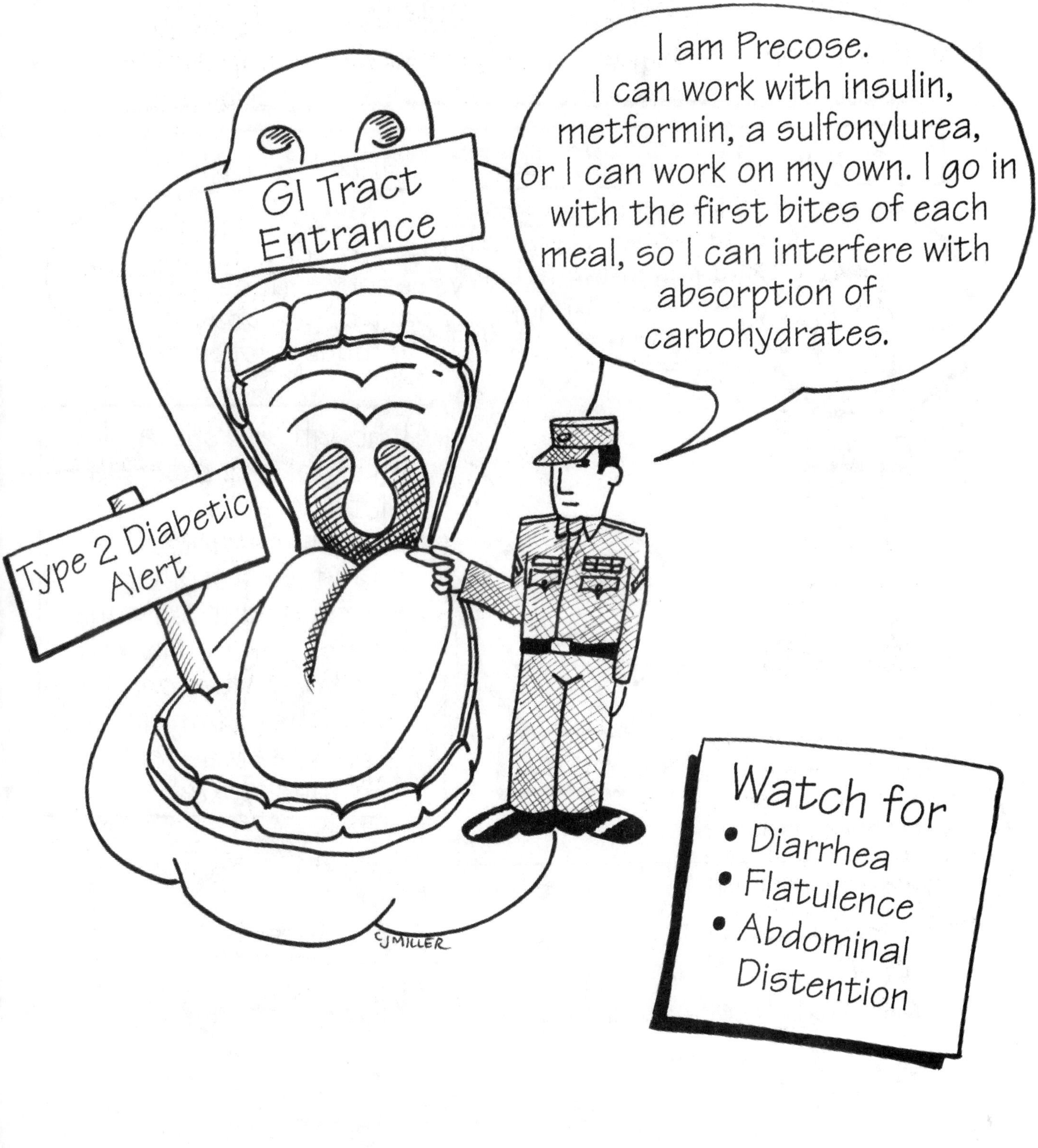
I am Precose.
I can work with insulin, metformin, a sulfonylurea, or I can work on my own. I go in with the first bites of each meal, so I can interfere with absorption of carbohydrates.
GI Tract Entrance
Type 2 Diabetic Alert
CJMILLER
Watch for
• Diarrhea
• Flatulence
• Abdominal Distention

Corticosteroids

Methylprednisolone (Solu-Medrol)
Dexamethasone (Decadron)
Prednisone (Deltasone)

Steroids... The Good, The Bad, and The Ugly!!!

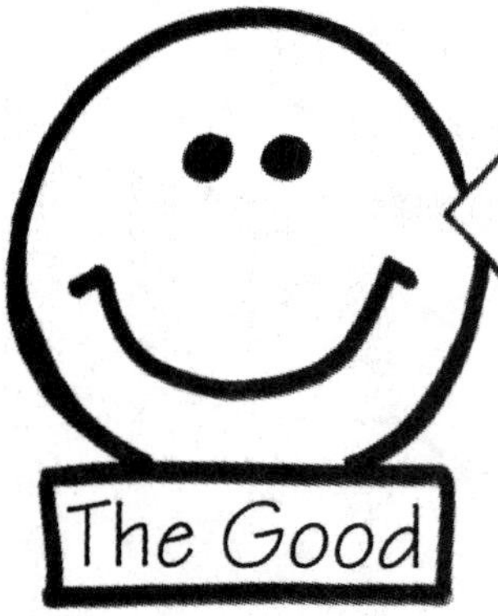

These drugs stop, control or reduce the inflammatory response, (local or systemic) in any part of the body by suppressing the immune system.

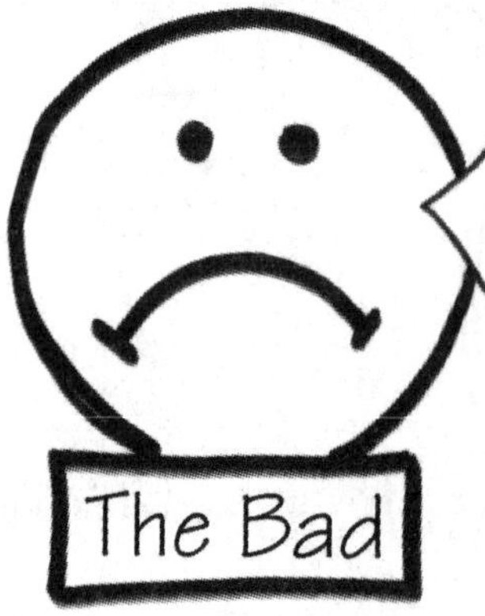

Although there is a slow internal and external deterioration of the body, the trade off is that the steroid in a chronic or autoimmune disorder will usually keep the body alive longer than if the inflammatory process was left unchecked.

The dose amount and duration of use dictate the extent of dependency and damage to the body. Watch for edema, peptic ulcers, delayed wound healing, osteoporosis & infections.

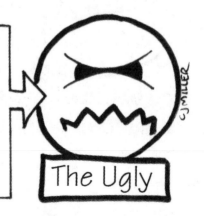

Glimepride (Amaryl) & Glipizide (Glucotrol)

"Amaryl and Glucotrol - Releasing Insulin from the Beta Cells."

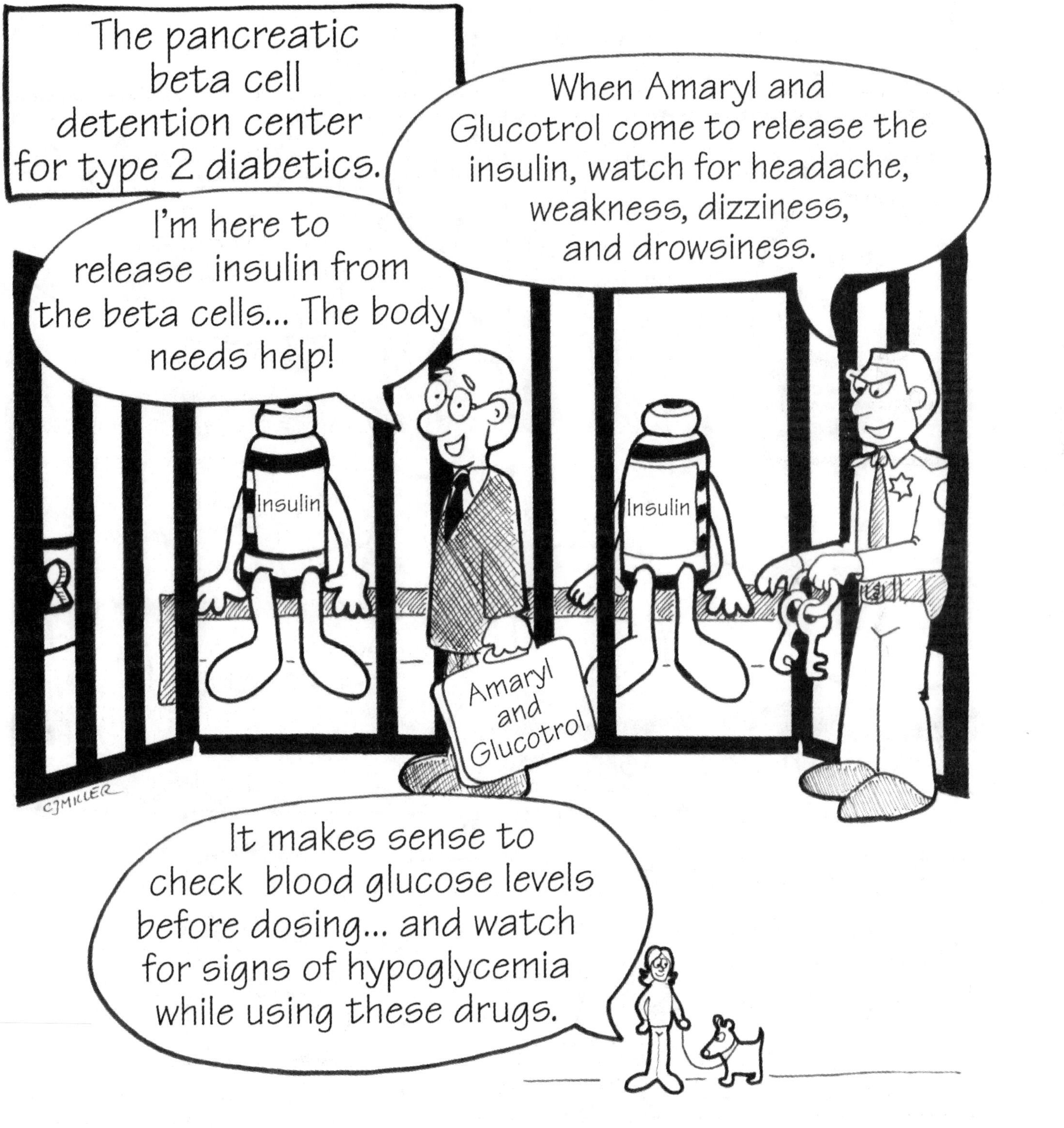

The pancreatic beta cell detention center for type 2 diabetics.
I'm here to release insulin from the beta cells... The body needs help!
When Amaryl and Glucotrol come to release the insulin, watch for headache, weakness, dizziness, and drowsiness.
Insulin
Insulin
Amaryl and Glucotrol
CJMILLER
It makes sense to check blood glucose levels before dosing... and watch for signs of hypoglycemia while using these drugs.

Glucagon

"Glucagon, When the Sugar's Gone!"

A first aid kit for severe hypoglycemia

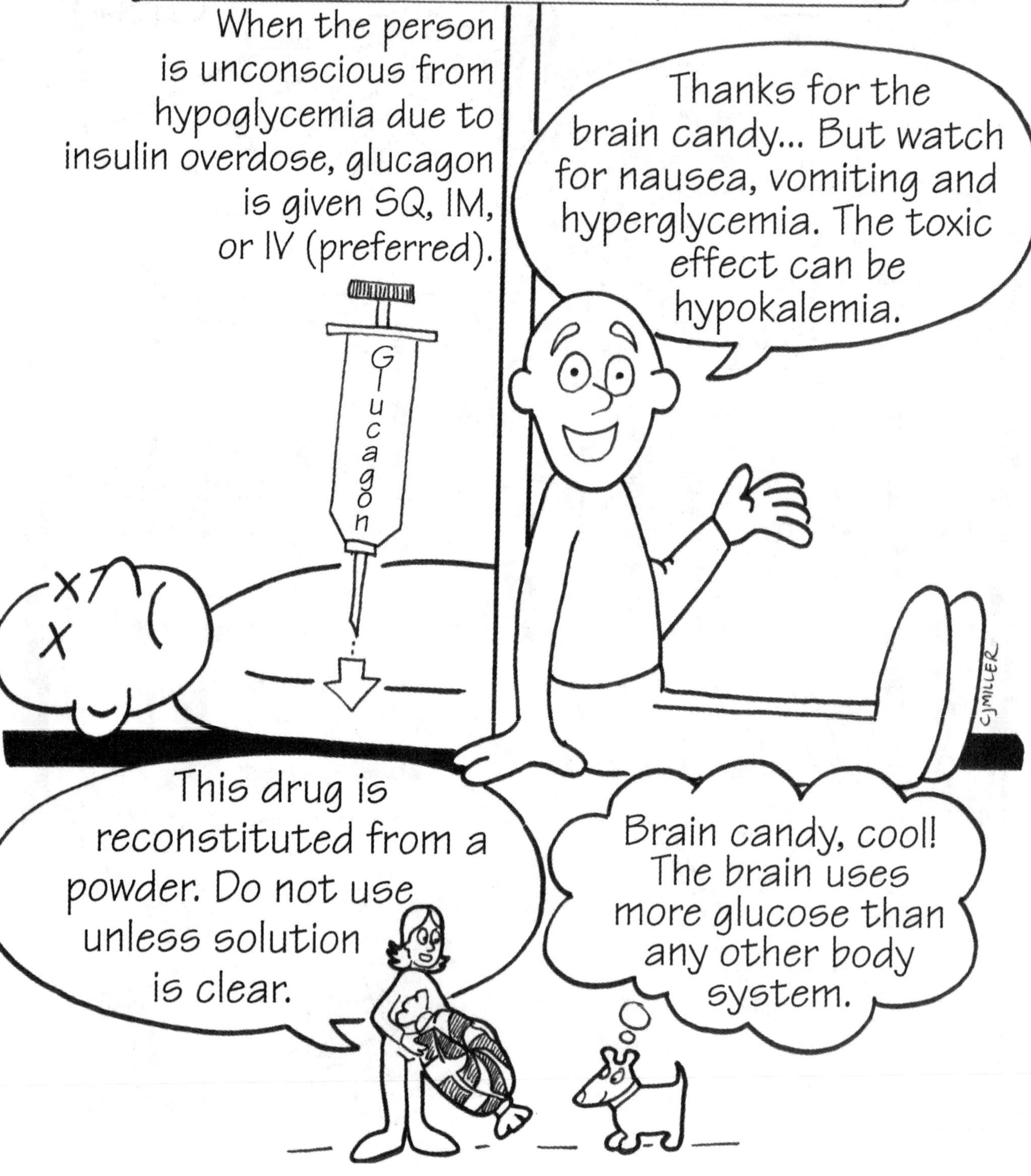
When the person is unconscious from hypoglycemia due to insulin overdose, glucagon is given SQ, IM, or IV (preferred).
Glucagon
Thanks for the brain candy... But watch for nausea, vomiting and hyperglycemia. The toxic effect can be hypokalemia.
CJMILLER
This drug is reconstituted from a powder. Do not use unless solution is clear.
Brain candy, cool! The brain uses more glucose than any other body system.

Insulin: Types, Onset, and Peaks

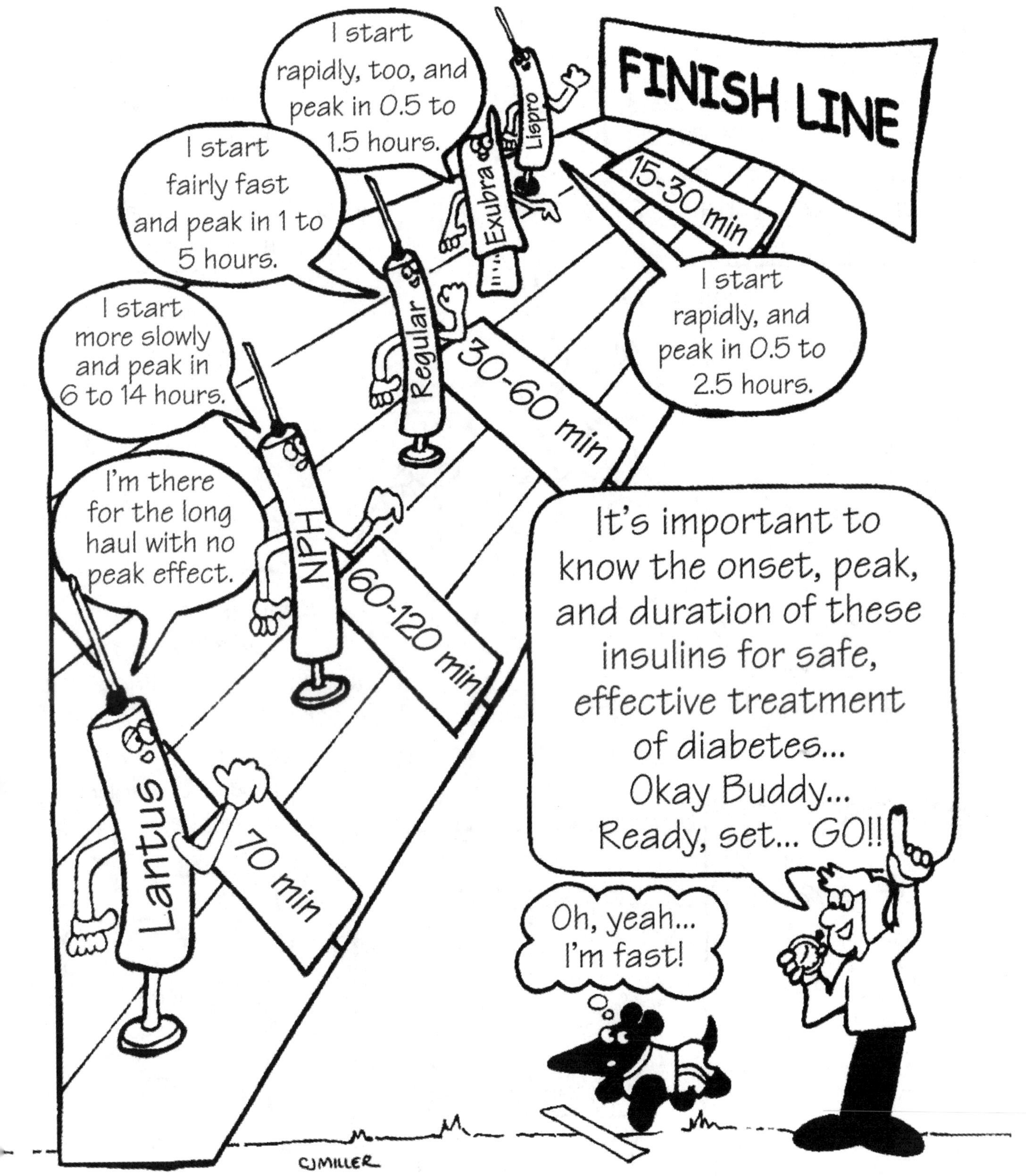
FINISH LINE
I start rapidly, too, and peak in 0.5 to 1.5 hours.
Lispro
Exubra
15-30 min
I start fairly fast and peak in 1 to 5 hours.
Regular
30-60 min
I start rapidly, and peak in 0.5 to 2.5 hours.
I start more slowly and peak in 6 to 14 hours.
NPH
60-120 min
I'm there for the long haul with no peak effect.
Lantus
70 min
It's important to know the onset, peak, and duration of these insulins for safe, effective treatment of diabetes... Okay Buddy... Ready, set... GO!!
Oh, yeah... I'm fast!
CJMILLER

Rapid Acting Insulin

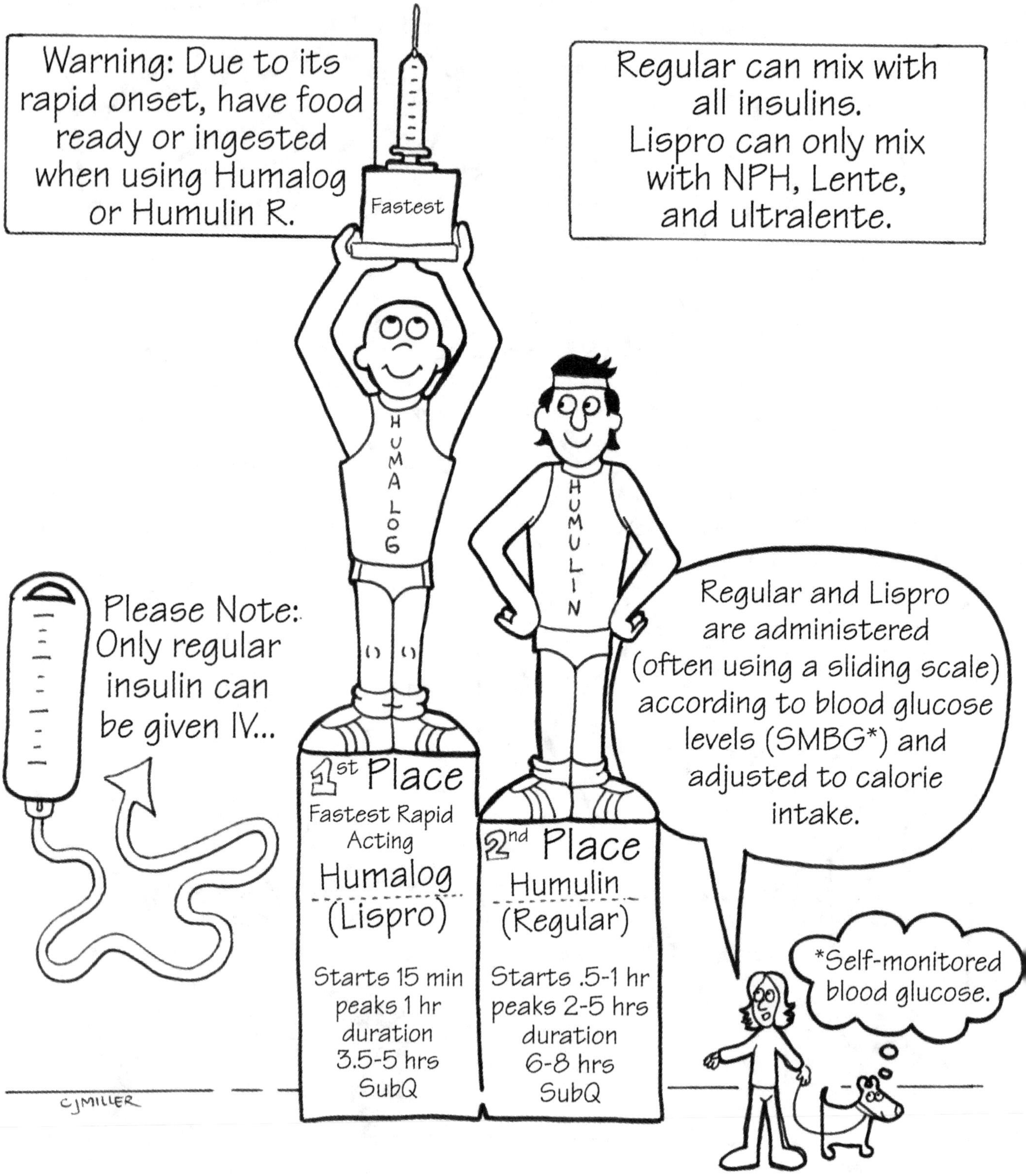
Warning: Due to its rapid onset, have food ready or ingested when using Humalog or Humulin R.
Fastest
Regular can mix with all insulins. Lispro can only mix with NPH, Lente, and ultralente.
HUMALOG
HUMULIN
Please Note: Only regular insulin can be given IV...
Regular and Lispro are administered (often using a sliding scale) according to blood glucose levels (SMBG*) and adjusted to calorie intake.
1st Place
Fastest Rapid Acting
Humalog
(Lispro)
Starts 15 min
peaks 1 hr
duration
3.5-5 hrs
SubQ
2nd Place
Humulin
(Regular)
Starts .5-1 hr
peaks 2-5 hrs
duration
6-8 hrs
SubQ
*Self-monitored blood glucose.
CJMILLER

Levothyroxine (Synthroid)

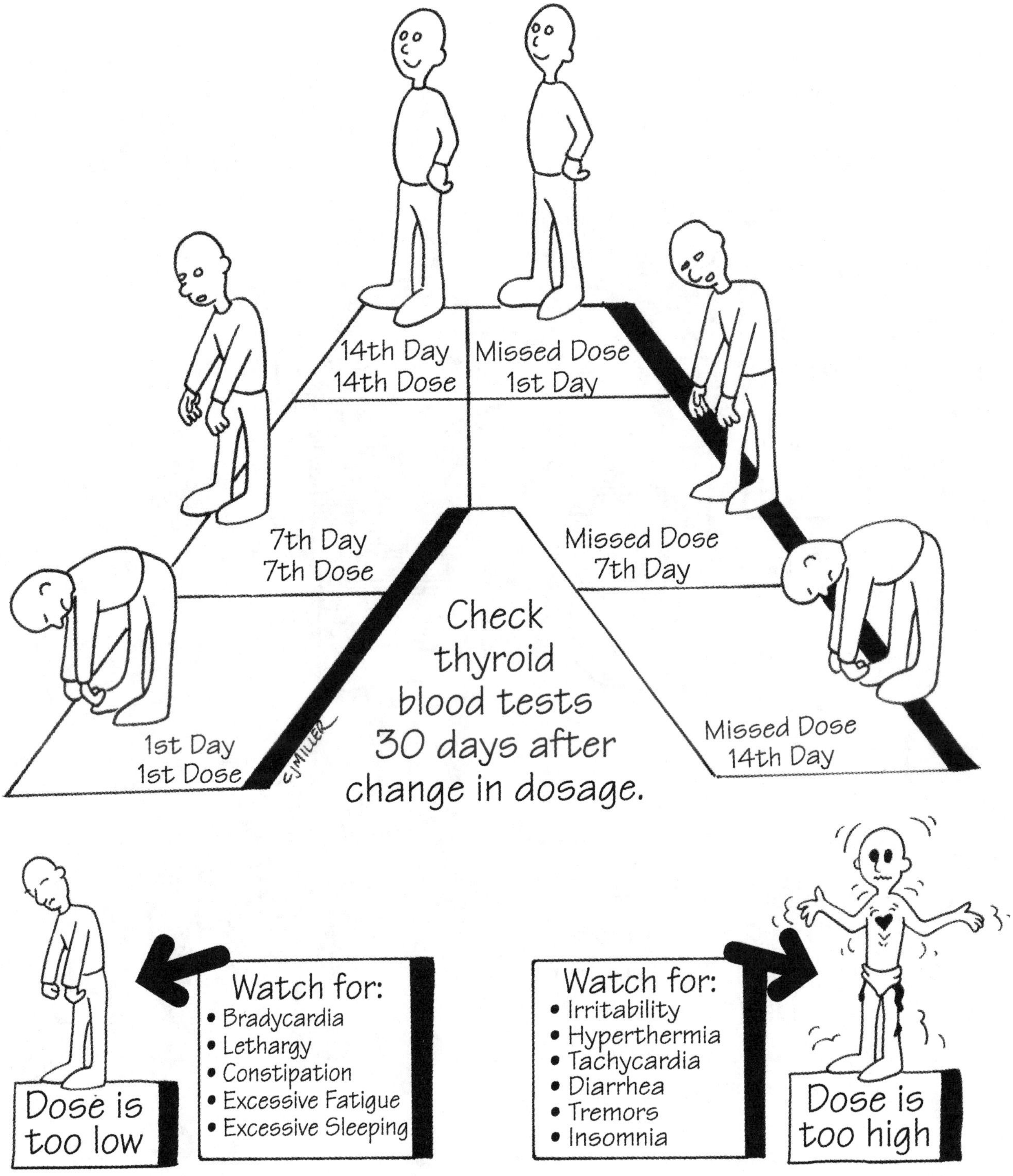
14th Day
14th Dose
Missed Dose
1st Day
7th Day
7th Dose
Missed Dose
7th Day
Check thyroid blood tests 30 days after change in dosage.
1st Day
1st Dose
Missed Dose
14th Day
CJMILLER
Dose is too low
Watch for:
• Bradycardia
• Lethargy
• Constipation
• Excessive Fatigue
• Excessive Sleeping
Watch for:
• Irritability
• Hyperthermia
• Tachycardia
• Diarrhea
• Tremors
• Insomnia
Dose is too high

Methimazole (Tapazole)

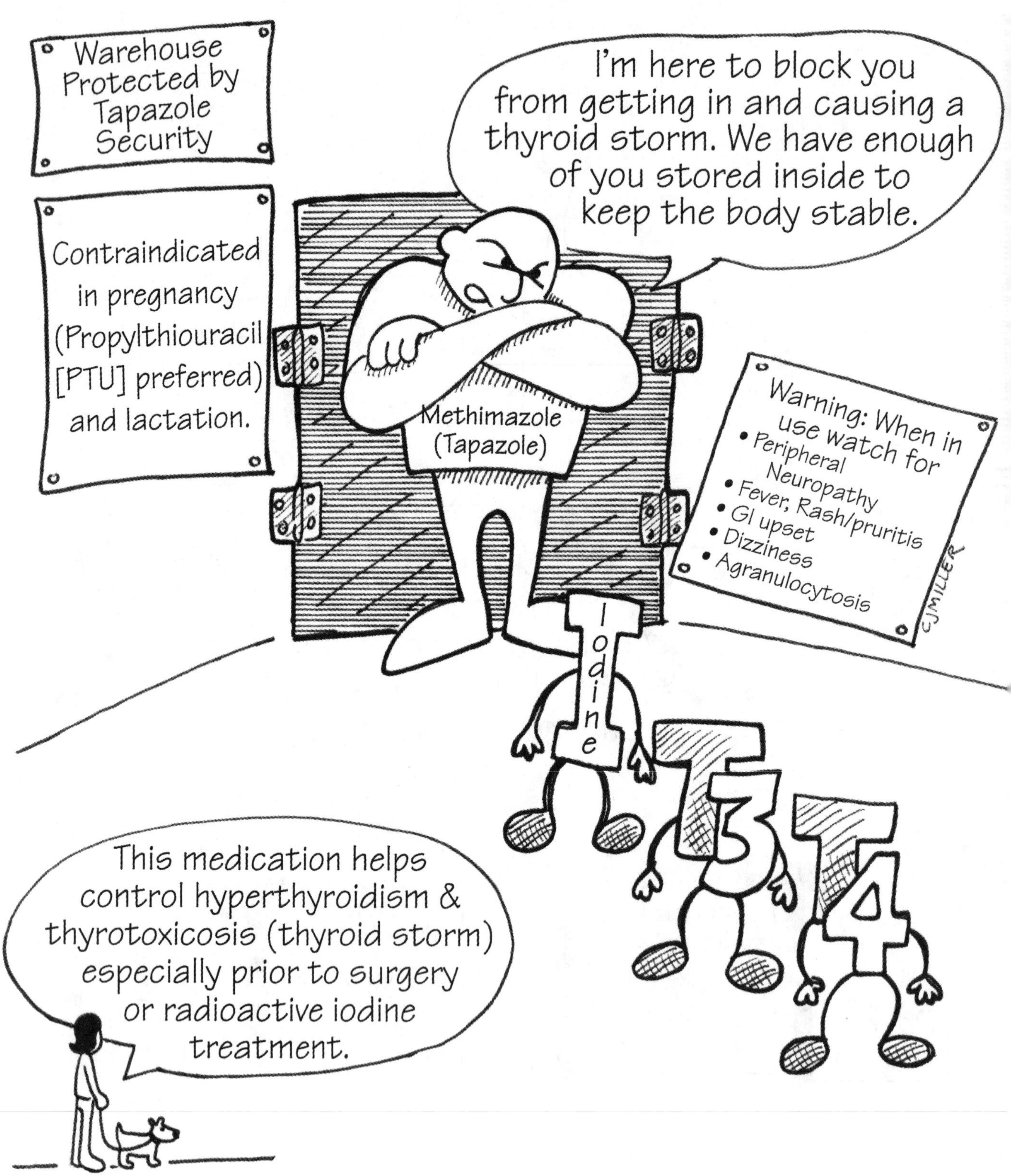

Warehouse Protected by Tapazole Security
Contraindicated in pregnancy (Propylthiouracil [PTU] preferred) and lactation.
I'm here to block you from getting in and causing a thyroid storm. We have enough of you stored inside to keep the body stable.
Methimazole (Tapazole)
Warning: When in use watch for
• Peripheral Neuropathy
• Fever, Rash/pruritis
• GI upset
• Dizziness
• Agranulocytosis
CJMILLER
Iodine
T3
T4
This medication helps control hyperthyroidism & thyrotoxicosis (thyroid storm) especially prior to surgery or radioactive iodine treatment.

Sulfonylureas

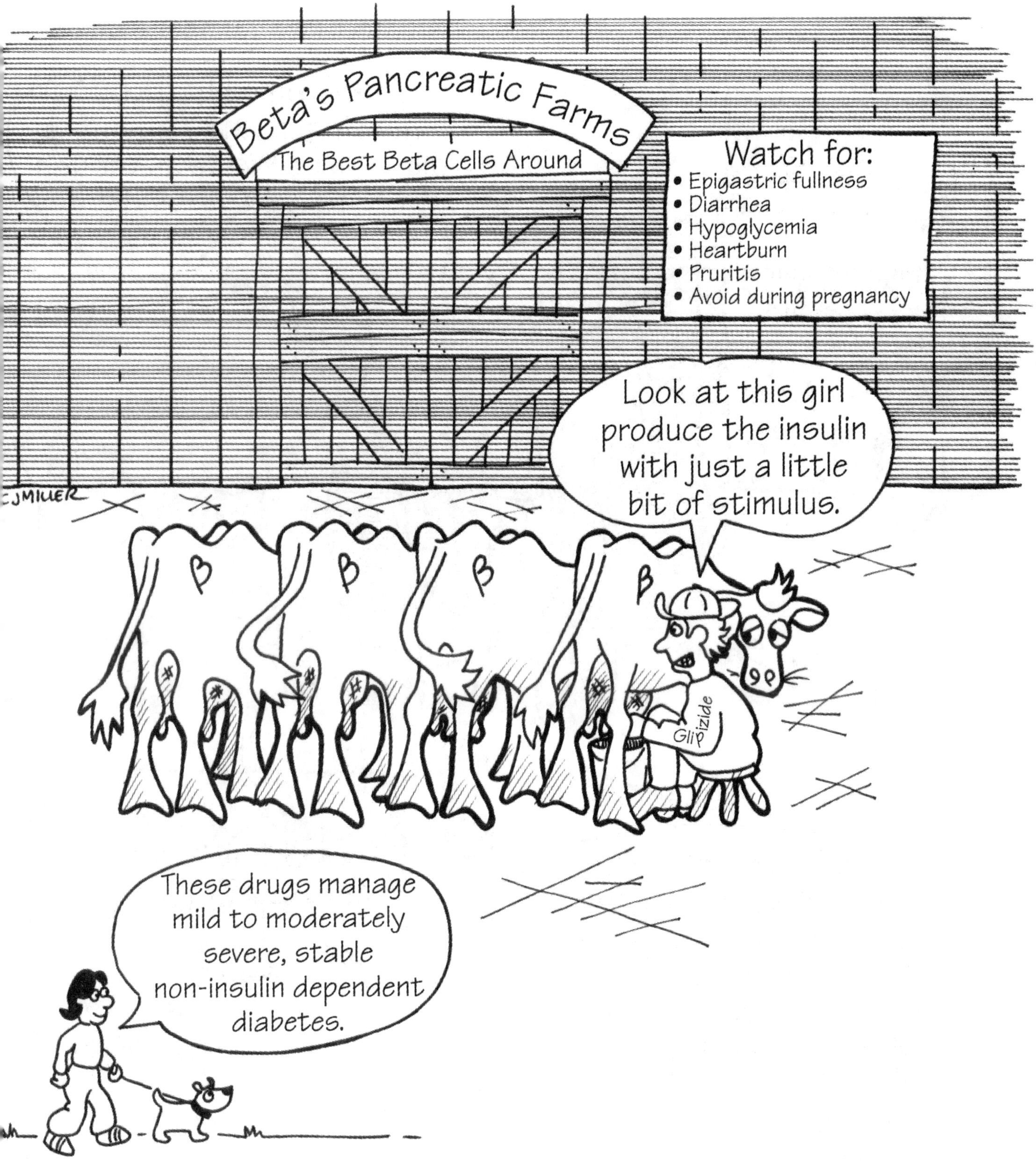
Beta's Pancreatic Farms
The Best Beta Cells Around
Watch for:
• Epigastric fullness
• Diarrhea
• Hypoglycemia
• Heartburn
• Pruritis
• Avoid during pregnancy
Look at this girl produce the insulin with just a little bit of stimulus.
Glipizide
These drugs manage mild to moderately severe, stable non-insulin dependent diabetes.
CJMILLER

Clopidogrel (Plavix)

"When Platelets Gather Together, Use Plavix for Crowd Control"

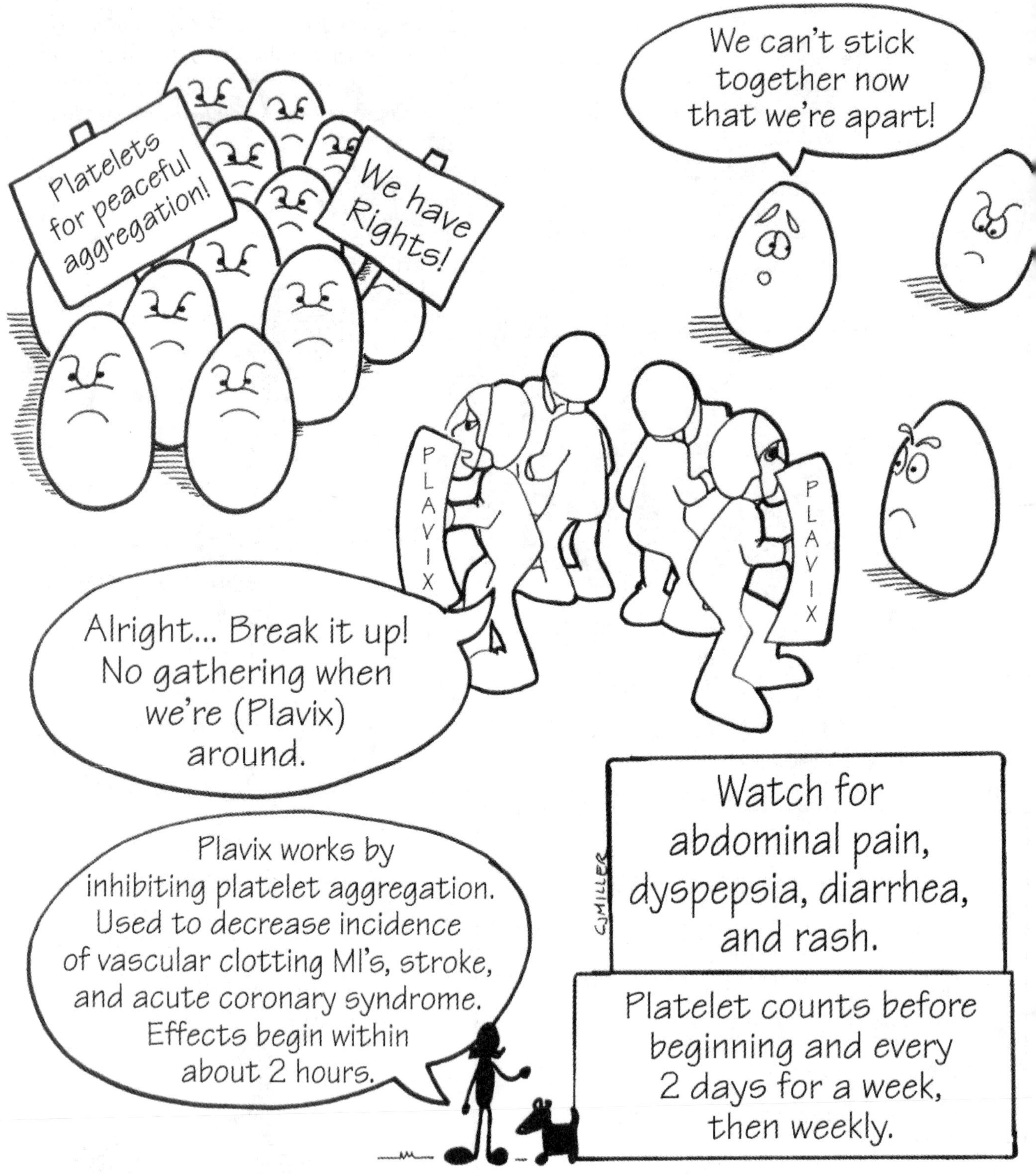
Platelets for peaceful aggregation!
We have Rights!
We can't stick together now that we're apart!
PLAVIX
PLAVIX
Alright... Break it up! No gathering when we're (Plavix) around.
Plavix works by inhibiting platelet aggregation. Used to decrease incidence of vascular clotting MI's, stroke, and acute coronary syndrome. Effects begin within about 2 hours.
Watch for abdominal pain, dyspepsia, diarrhea, and rash.
Platelet counts before beginning and every 2 days for a week, then weekly.
CJMILLER

Epoetin Alfa (Procrit)

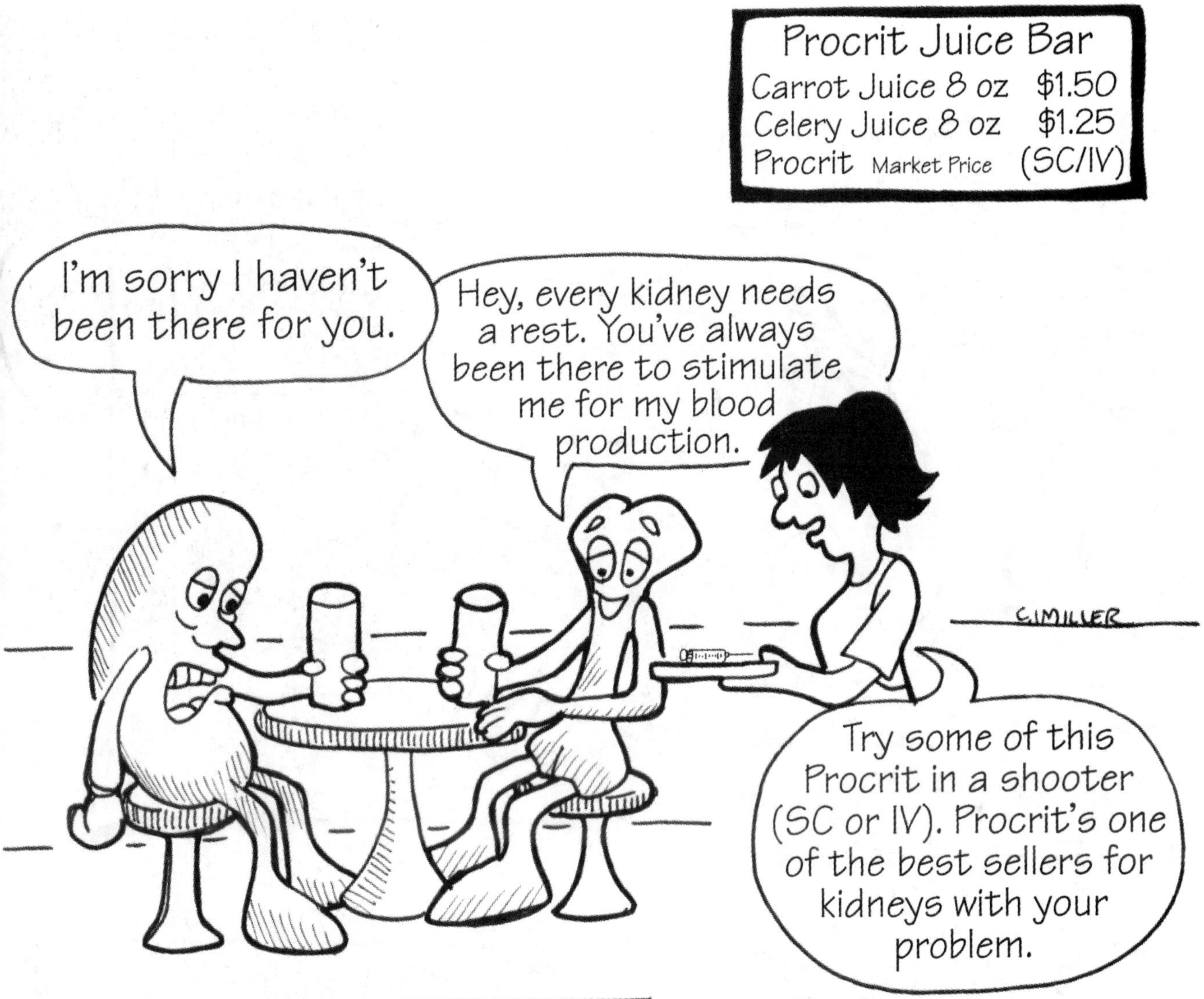
Procrit Juice Bar
Carrot Juice 8 oz $1.50
Celery Juice 8 oz $1.25
Procrit Market Price (SC/IV)
I'm sorry I haven't been there for you.
Hey, every kidney needs a rest. You've always been there to stimulate me for my blood production.
Try some of this Procrit in a shooter (SC or IV). Procrit's one of the best sellers for kidneys with your problem.
C.MILLER

Procrit is synthetic erythropoietin, which increases Hct and Hgb. Used to treat anemia associated with renal failure and chemotherapy. Watch for hypertension, headache, nausea.

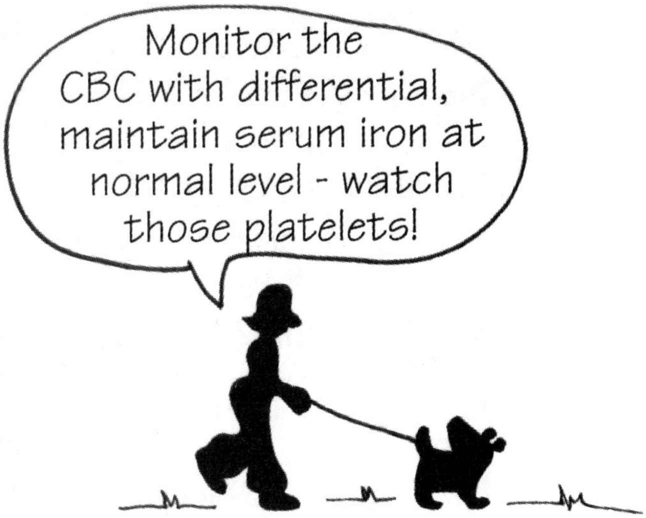
Monitor the CBC with differential, maintain serum iron at normal level - watch those platelets!

Heparin

The Clotting Round-Up

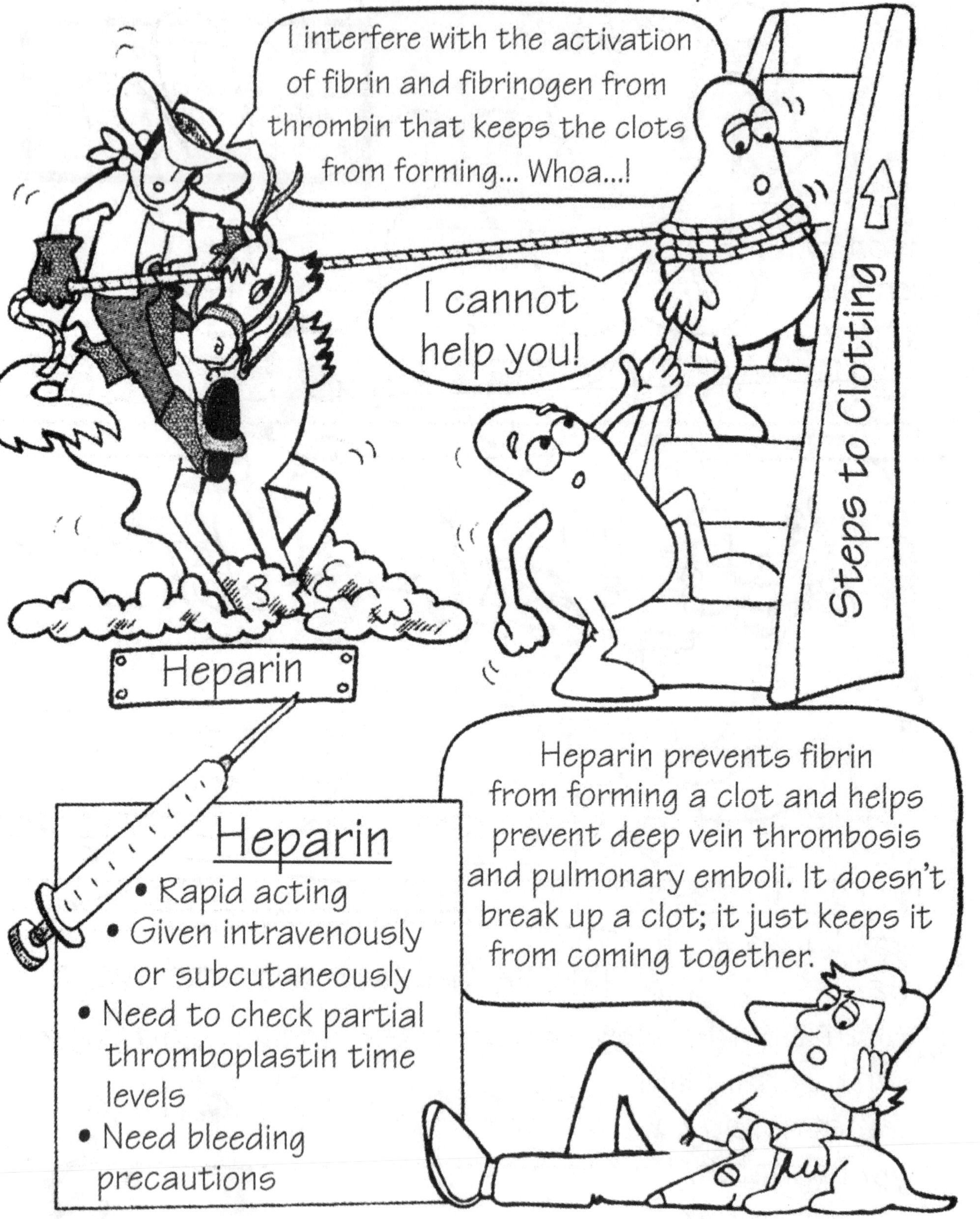
I interfere with the activation of fibrin and fibrinogen from thrombin that keeps the clots from forming... Whoa...!
I cannot help you!
Steps to Clotting
Heparin
Heparin
• Rapid acting
• Given intravenously or subcutaneously
• Need to check partial thromboplastin time levels
• Need bleeding precautions
Heparin prevents fibrin from forming a clot and helps prevent deep vein thrombosis and pulmonary emboli. It doesn't break up a clot; it just keeps it from coming together.

Heparin - Coumadin Tests

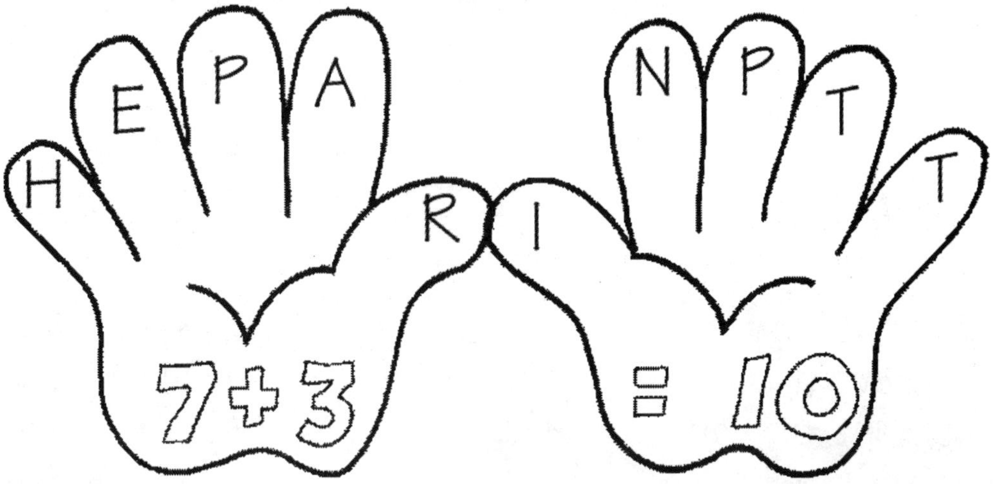

HEPARIN + PTT = 10 LETTERS

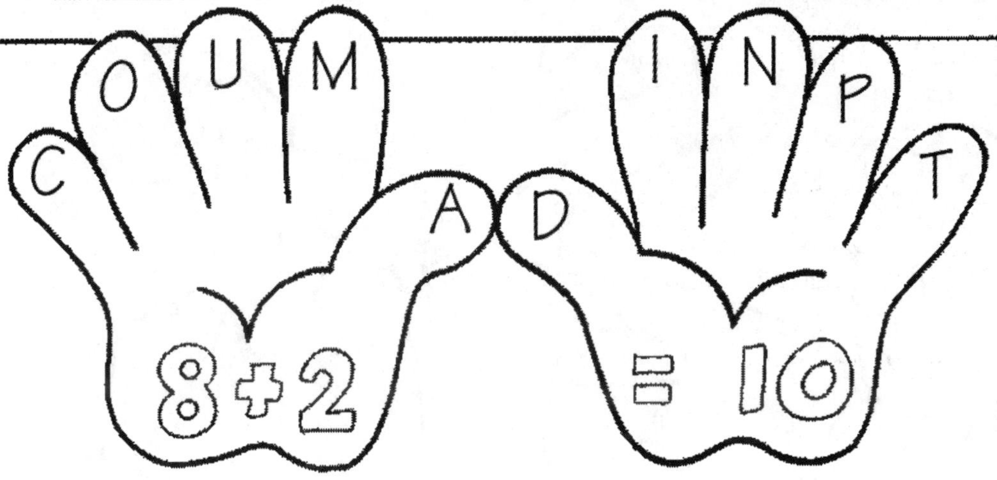

COUMADIN + PT = 10 LETTERS

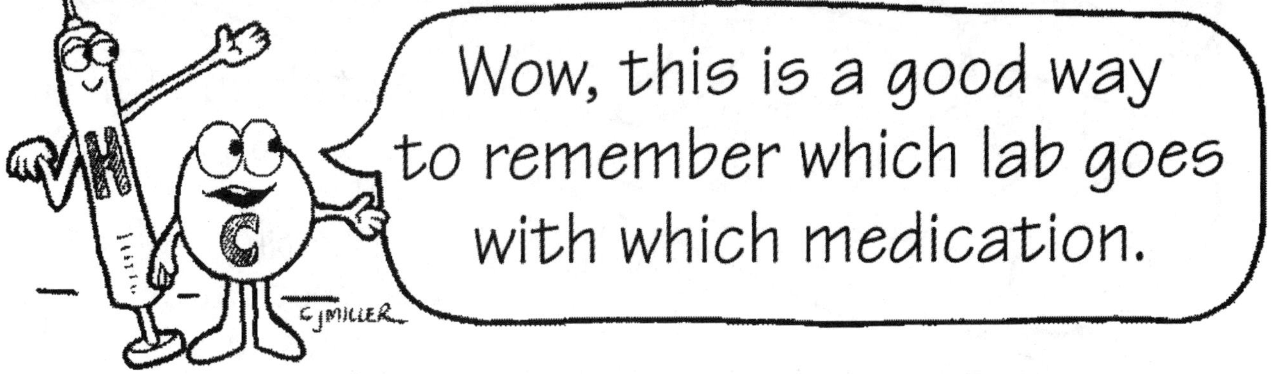
Wow, this is a good way to remember which lab goes with which medication.
H
C
CJMILLER

Iron Supplements

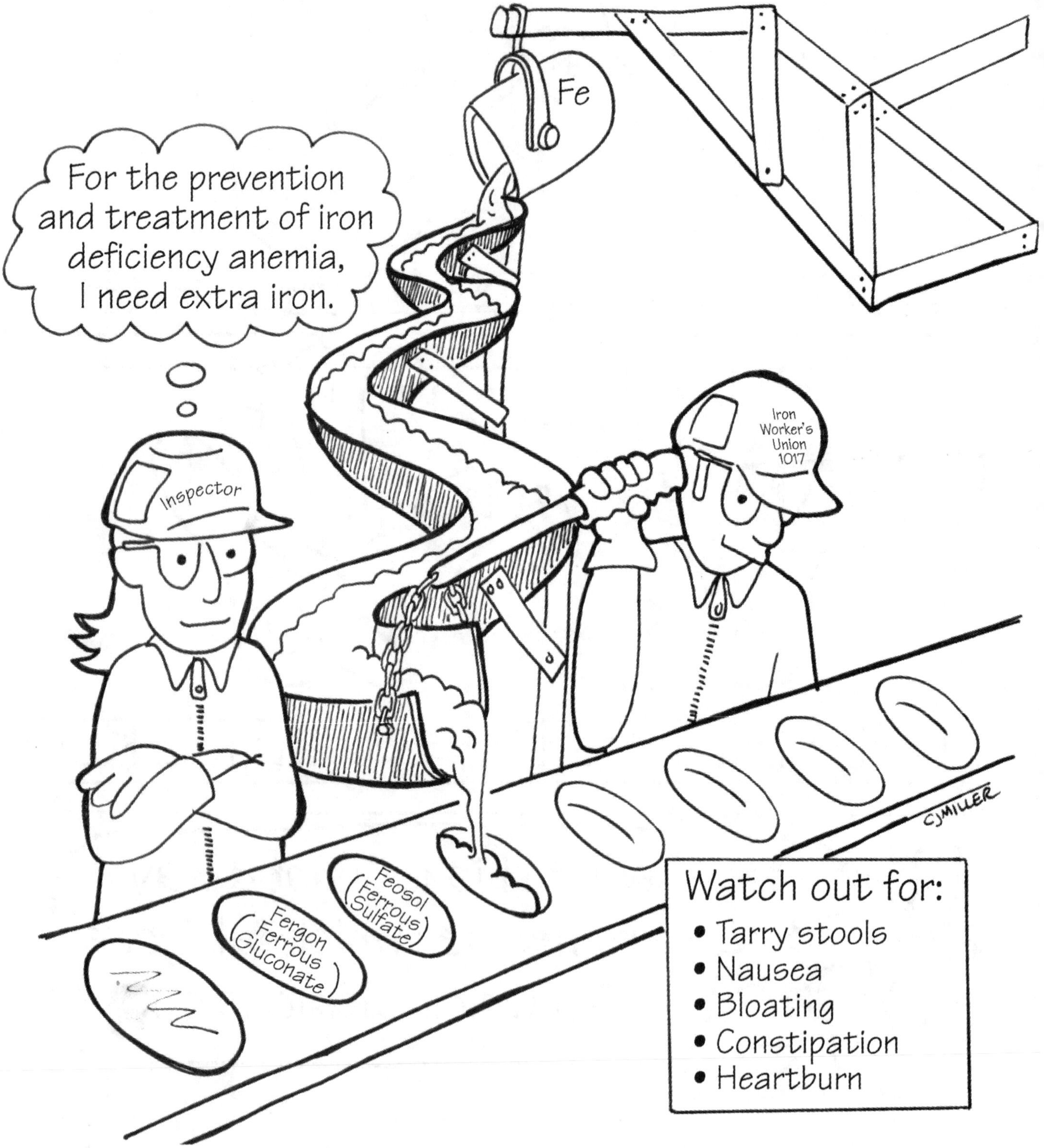

Watch out for:

- Tarry stools
- Nausea
- Bloating
- Constipation
- Heartburn

Thrombolytics

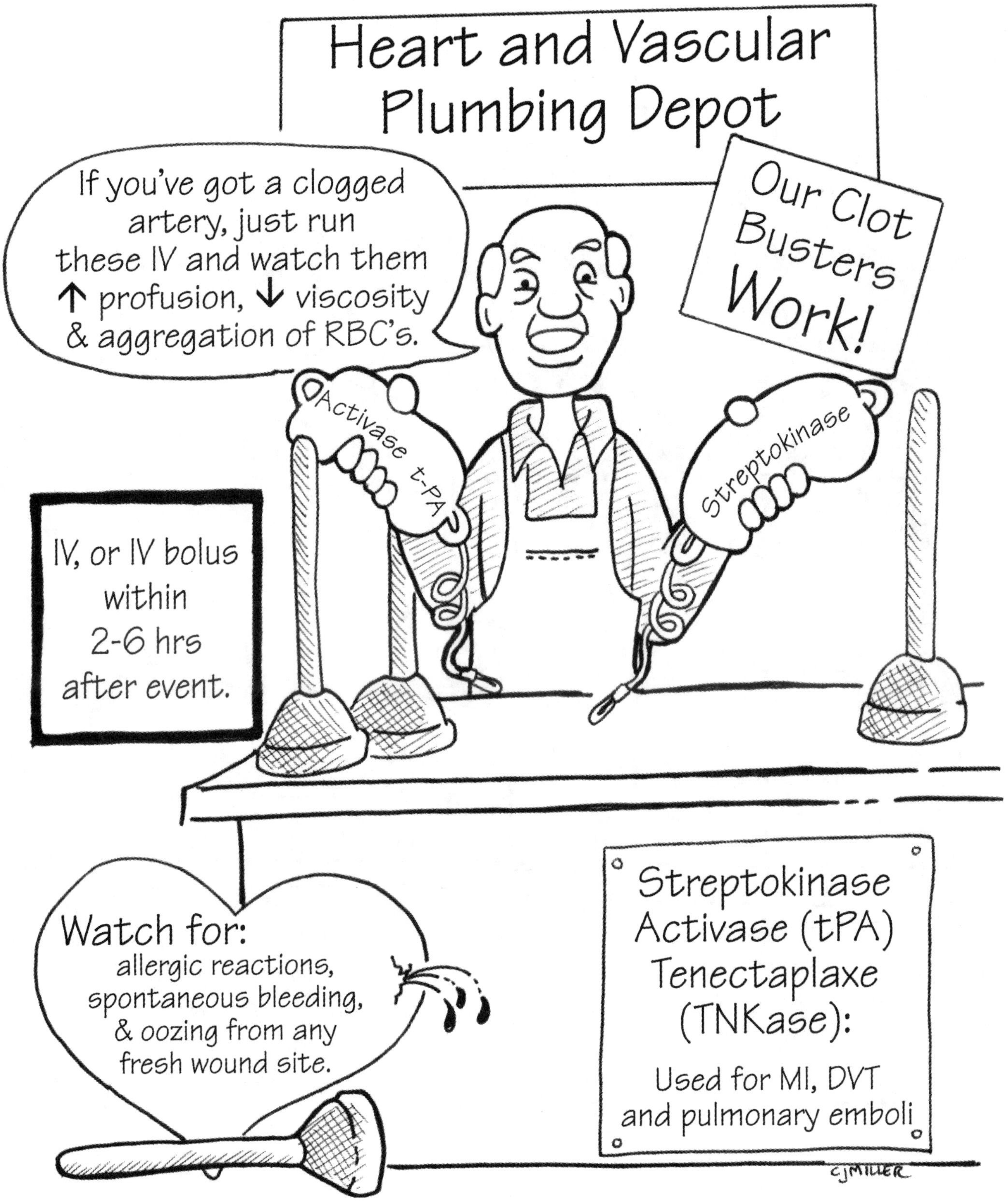

Heart and Vascular Plumbing Depot
If you've got a clogged artery, just run these IV and watch them ↑ profusion, ↓ viscosity & aggregation of RBC's.
Our Clot Busters Work!
Activase t-PA
Streptokinase
IV, or IV bolus within 2-6 hrs after event.
Watch for: allergic reactions, spontaneous bleeding, & oozing from any fresh wound site.
Streptokinase Activase (tPA) Tenectaplaxe (TNKase): Used for MI, DVT and pulmonary emboli
CJMILLER

Warfarin (Coumadin)

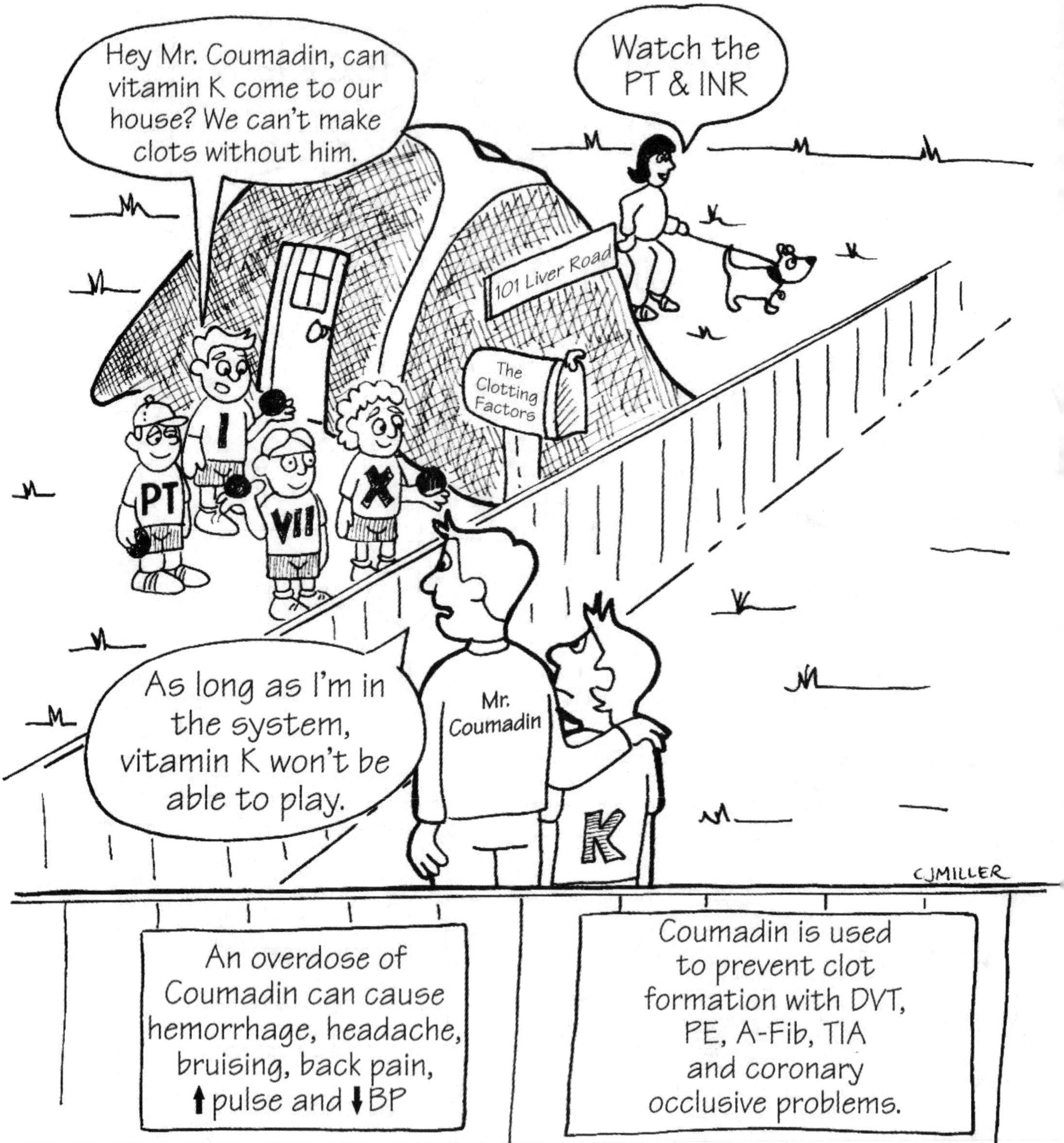
Hey Mr. Coumadin, can vitamin K come to our house? We can't make clots without him.
Watch the PT & INR
101 Liver Road
The Clotting Factors
PT
I
VII
X
As long as I'm in the system, vitamin K won't be able to play.
Mr. Coumadin
K
CJMILLER
An overdose of Coumadin can cause hemorrhage, headache, bruising, back pain, ↑ pulse and ↓ BP
Coumadin is used to prevent clot formation with DVT, PE, A-Fib, TIA and coronary occlusive problems.

Analgesics

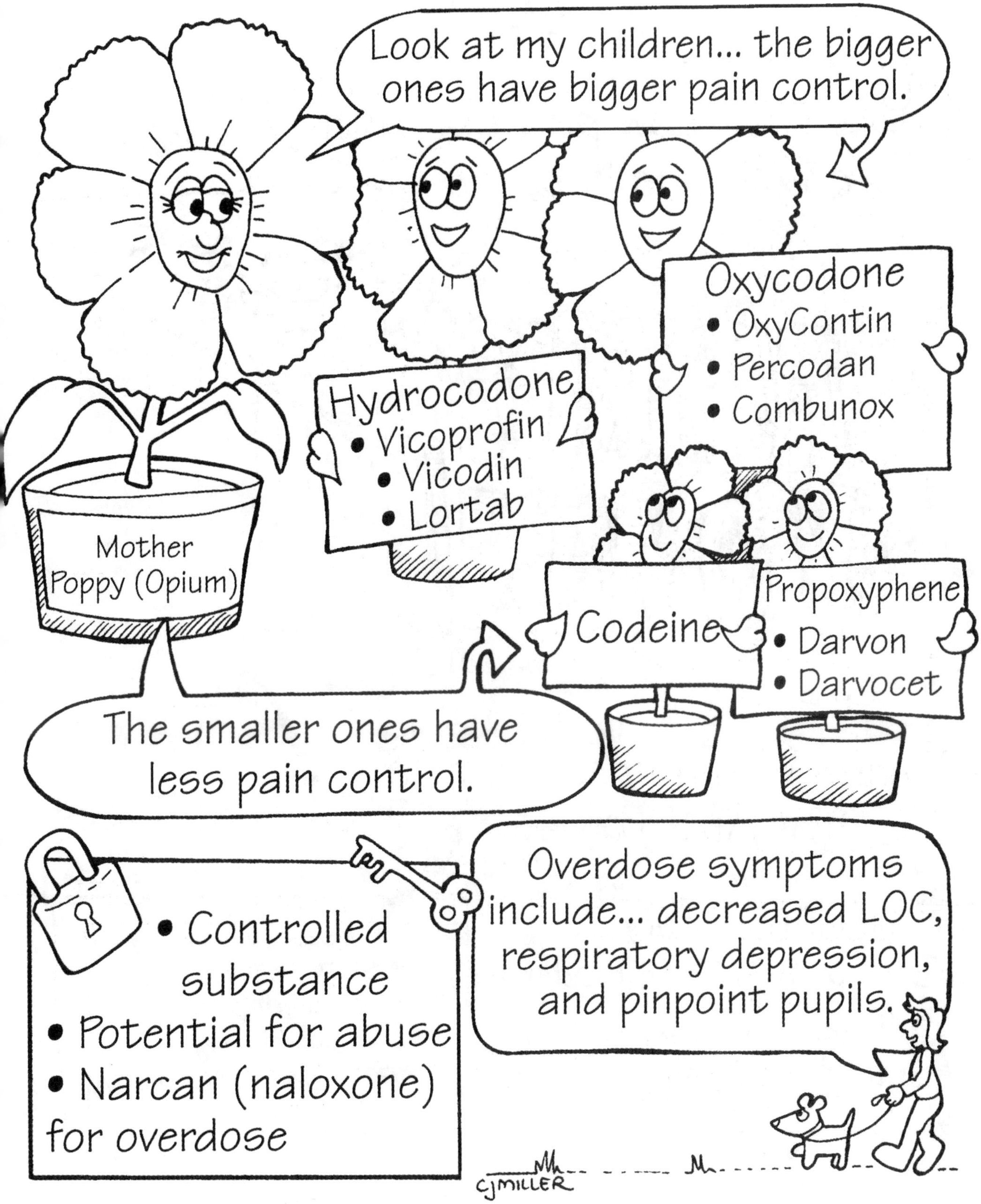

Look at my children... the bigger ones have bigger pain control.
Hydrocodone
• Vicoprofin
• Vicodin
• Lortab
Oxycodone
• OxyContin
• Percodan
• Combunox
Mother Poppy (Opium)
Codeine
Propoxyphene
• Darvon
• Darvocet
The smaller ones have less pain control.
• Controlled substance
• Potential for abuse
• Narcan (naloxone) for overdose
Overdose symptoms include... decreased LOC, respiratory depression, and pinpoint pupils.
CJMILLER

Aspirin

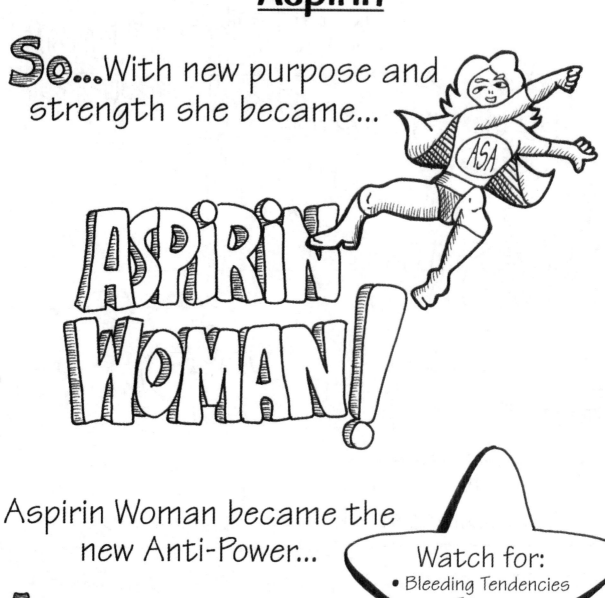

So... With new purpose and strength she became...

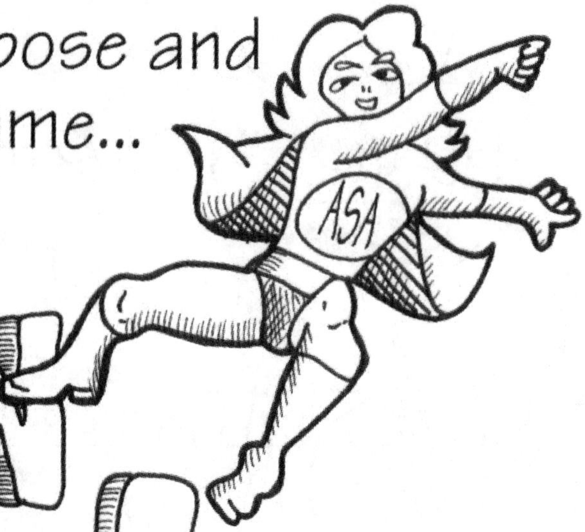

ASPIRIN WOMAN!

Aspirin Woman became the new Anti-Power...

Anti-inflammatory
Anti-pain (mild to moderate)
Anti-pyretic
Anti-platelet aggregation

Watch for:

- Bleeding Tendencies
- Tinnitus
- Stomach Pain
- Thrombocytopenia

CJMILLER

Morphine

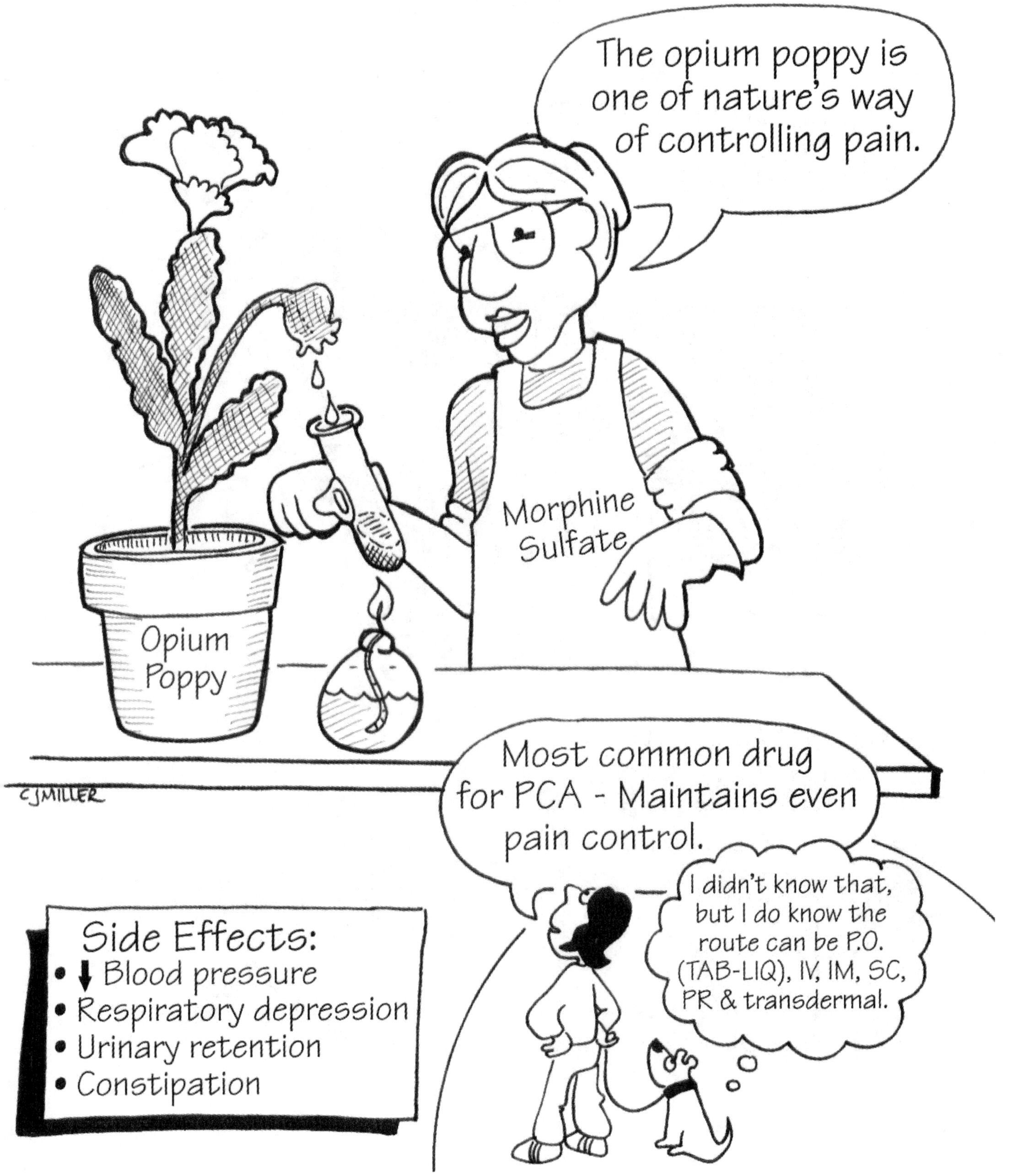

The opium poppy is one of nature's way of controlling pain.
Morphine Sulfate
Opium Poppy
CJMILLER
Most common drug for PCA - Maintains even pain control.
I didn't know that, but I do know the route can be P.O. (TAB-LIQ), IV, IM, SC, PR & transdermal.
Side Effects:
• ↓ Blood pressure
• Respiratory depression
• Urinary retention
• Constipation

Naloxone (Narcan)

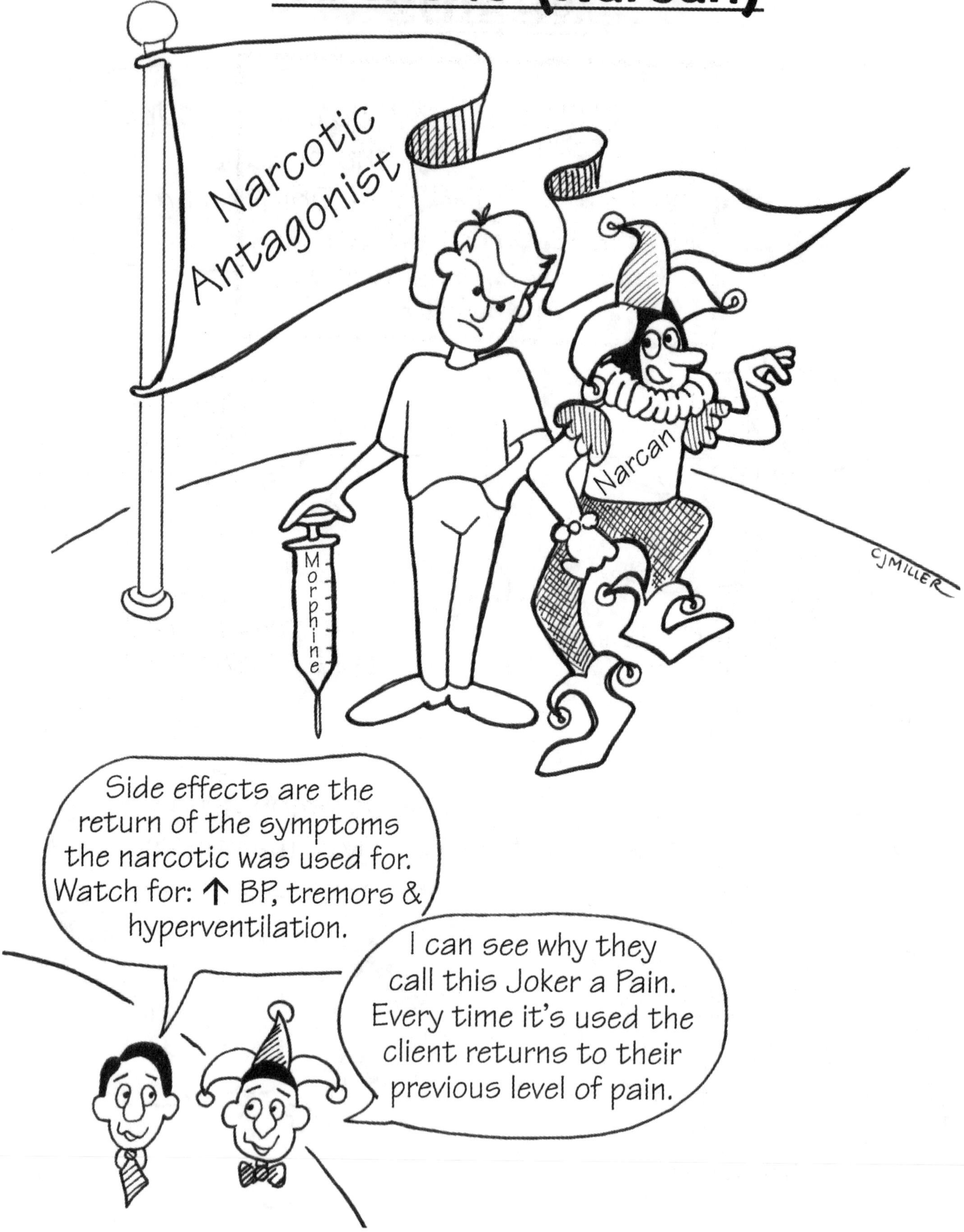

Narcotic Antagonist
Narcan
Morphine
CJMILLER
Side effects are the return of the symptoms the narcotic was used for. Watch for: ↑ BP, tremors & hyperventilation.
I can see why they call this Joker a Pain. Every time it's used the client returns to their previous level of pain.

NSAIDs

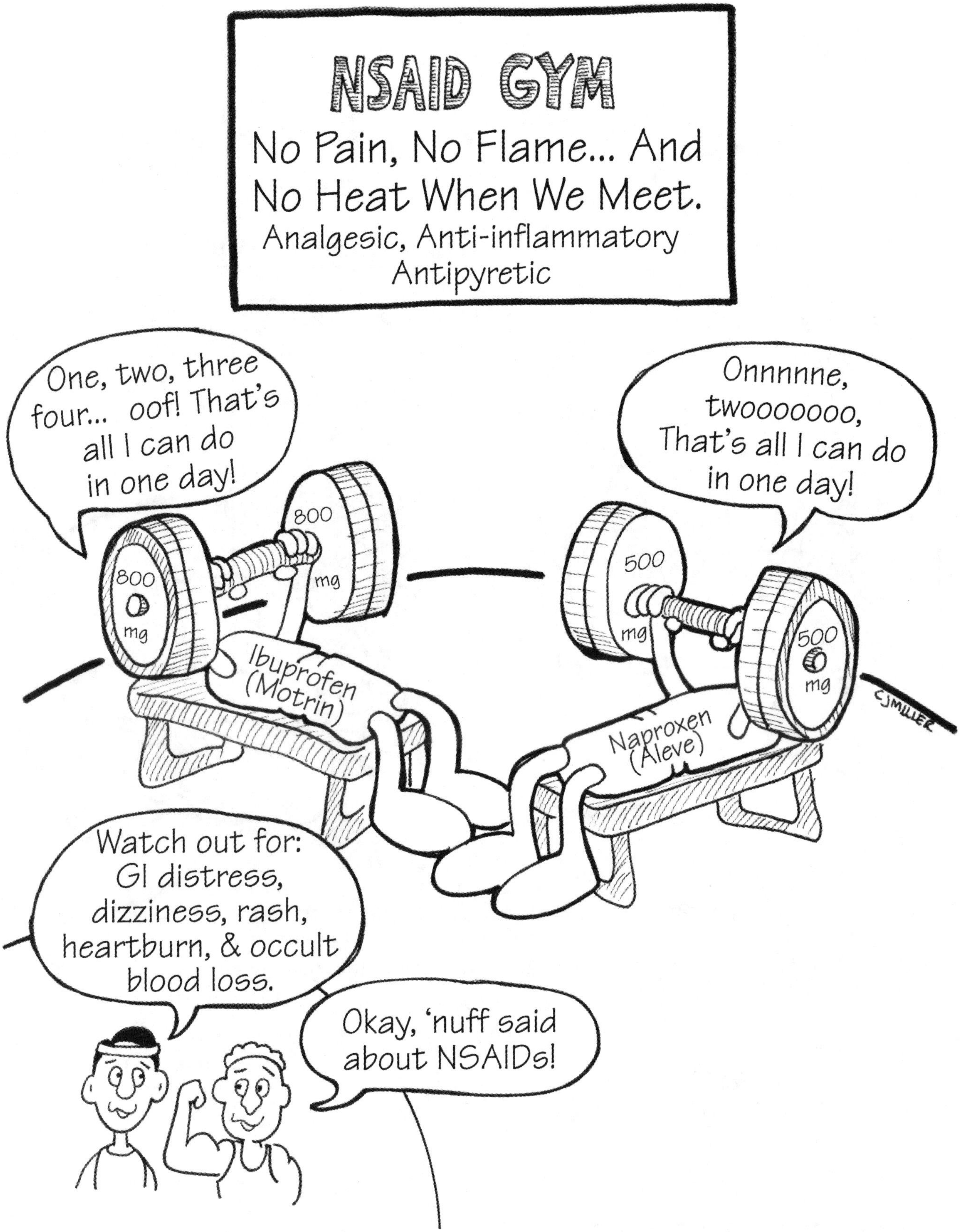
NSAID GYM
No Pain, No Flame... And No Heat When We Meet.
Analgesic, Anti-inflammatory Antipyretic
One, two, three four... oof! That's all I can do in one day!
Onnnnne, twooooooo, That's all I can do in one day!
800 mg
800 mg
Ibuprofen (Motrin)
500 mg
500 mg
Naproxen (Aleve)
CJMILLER
Watch out for: GI distress, dizziness, rash, heartburn, & occult blood loss.
Okay, 'nuff said about NSAIDs!

Antiepileptic Agents

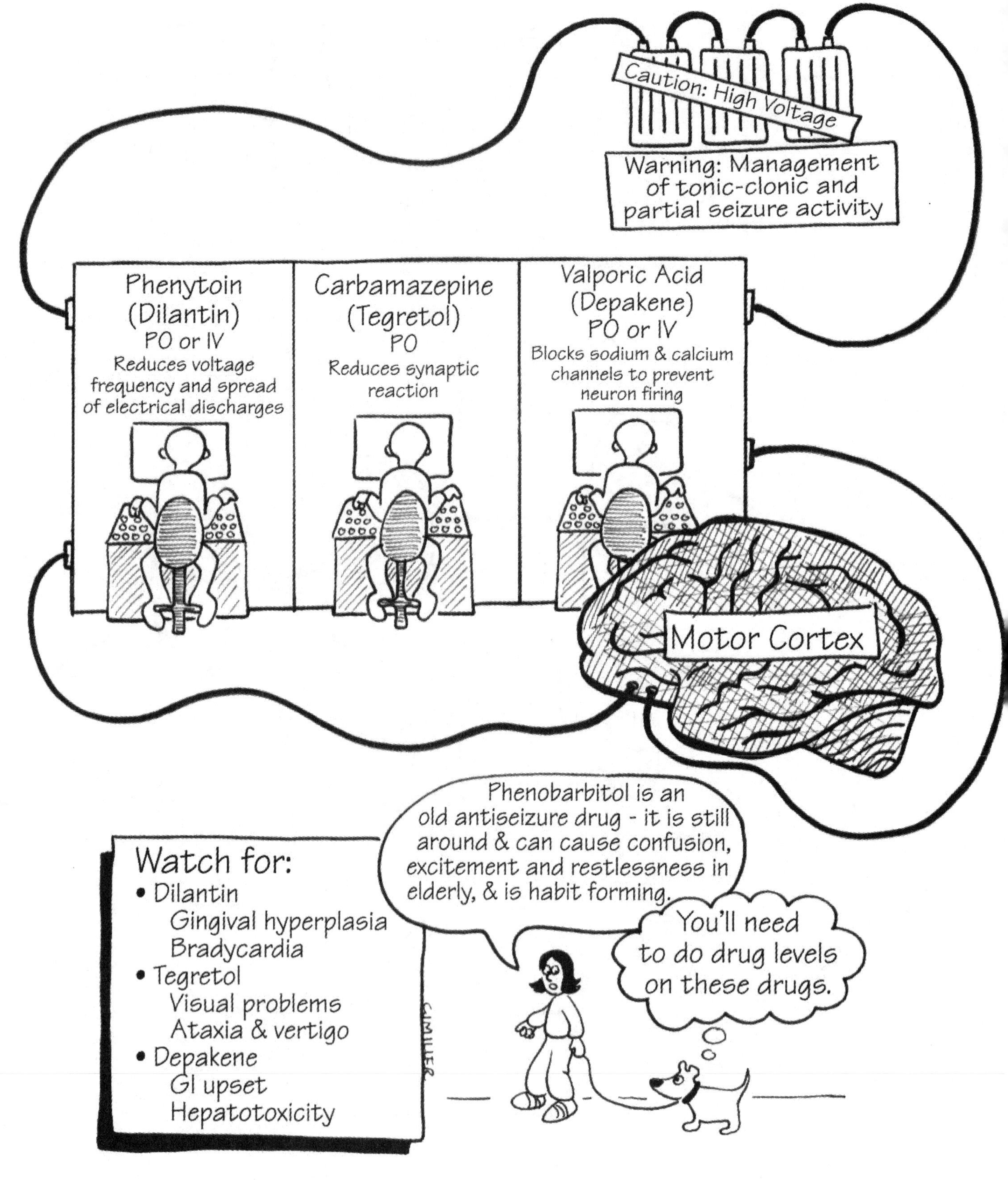

Caution: High Voltage
Warning: Management of tonic-clonic and partial seizure activity
Phenytoin (Dilantin) PO or IV Reduces voltage frequency and spread of electrical discharges
Carbamazepine (Tegretol) PO Reduces synaptic reaction
Valporic Acid (Depakene) PO or IV Blocks sodium & calcium channels to prevent neuron firing
Motor Cortex
Phenobarbitol is an old antiseizure drug - it is still around & can cause confusion, excitement and restlessness in elderly, & is habit forming.
You'll need to do drug levels on these drugs.
Watch for:
• Dilantin
Gingival hyperplasia
Bradycardia
• Tegretol
Visual problems
Ataxia & vertigo
• Depakene
GI upset
Hepatotoxicity

Benztropine (Cogentin)

"Controlling The Uncontrollable"

Anticholinergic; Antiparkinson Drug

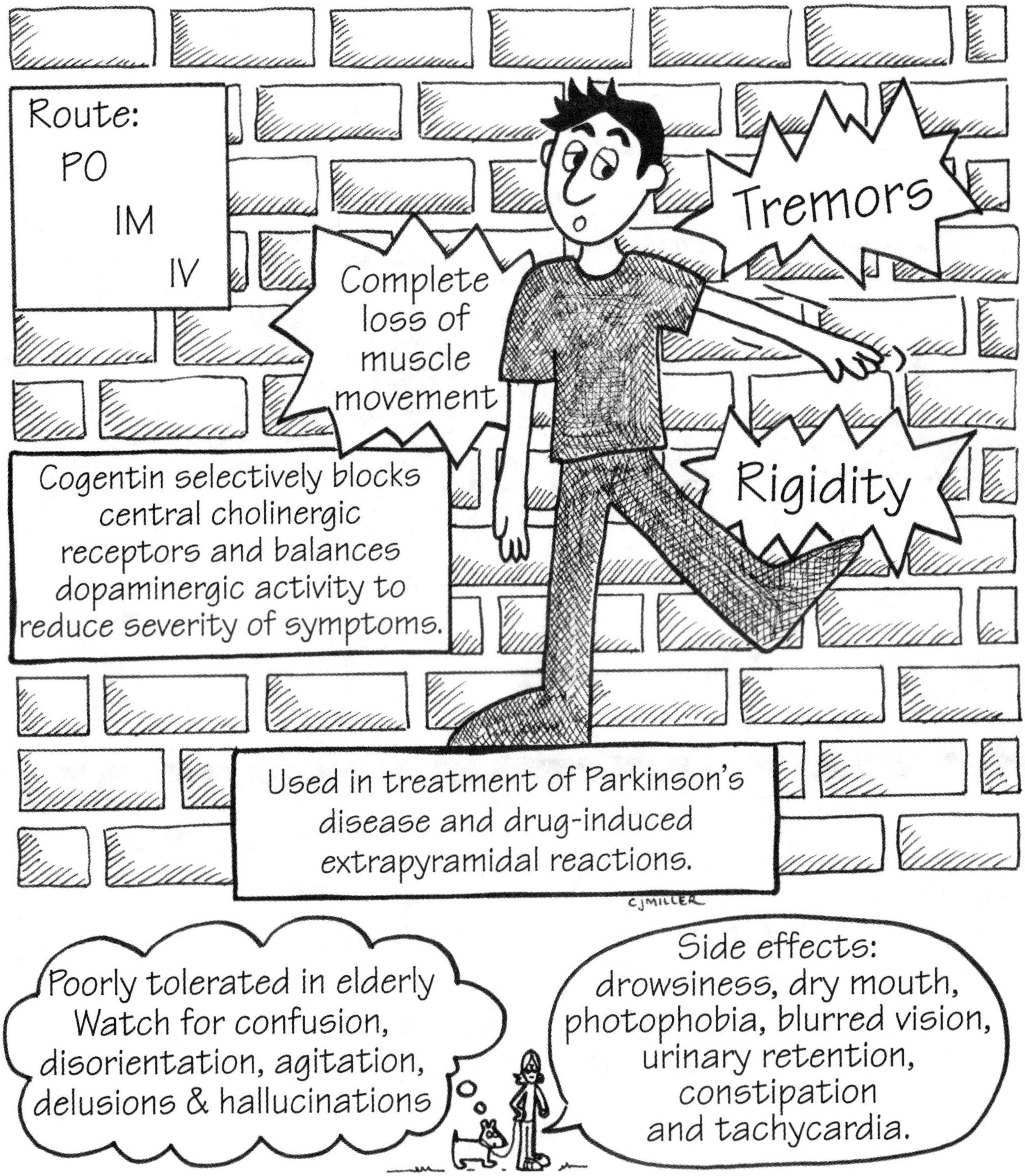

Route:
PO
IM
IV
Tremors
Complete loss of muscle movement
Rigidity
Cogentin selectively blocks central cholinergic receptors and balances dopaminergic activity to reduce severity of symptoms.
Used in treatment of Parkinson's disease and drug-induced extrapyramidal reactions.
CJMILLER
Poorly tolerated in elderly Watch for confusion, disorientation, agitation, delusions & hallucinations
Side effects: drowsiness, dry mouth, photophobia, blurred vision, urinary retention, constipation and tachycardia.

Carbamazepine (Tegretol)

"Stop the Seizures Before They Start"

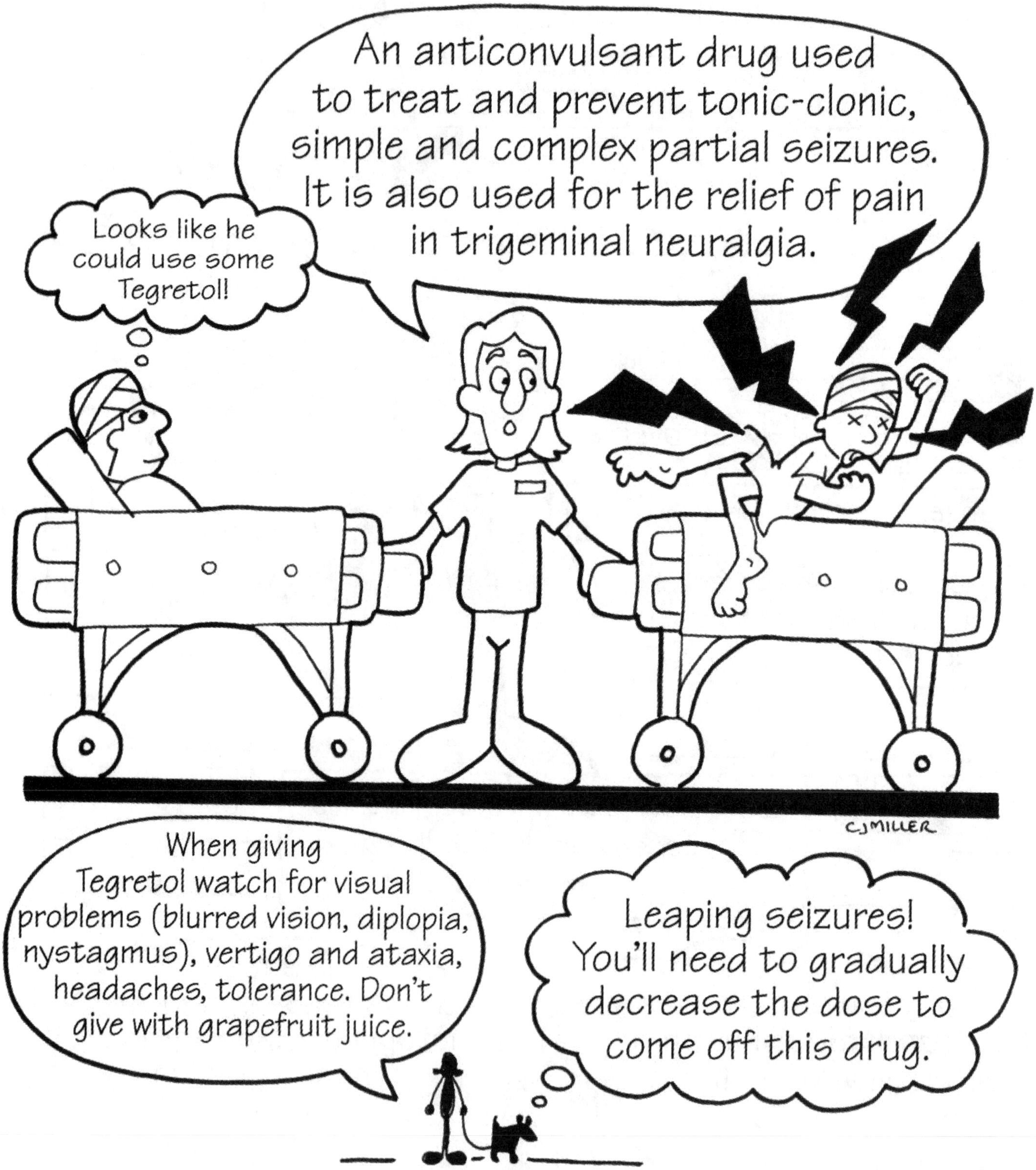
Looks like he could use some Tegretol!
An anticonvulsant drug used to treat and prevent tonic-clonic, simple and complex partial seizures. It is also used for the relief of pain in trigeminal neuralgia.
CJMILLER
When giving Tegretol watch for visual problems (blurred vision, diplopia, nystagmus), vertigo and ataxia, headaches, tolerance. Don't give with grapefruit juice.
Leaping seizures! You'll need to gradually decrease the dose to come off this drug.

Clonazepam (Klonopin)

"Benzodiazepine and Anticonvulsant...
...Two sides to the Story."

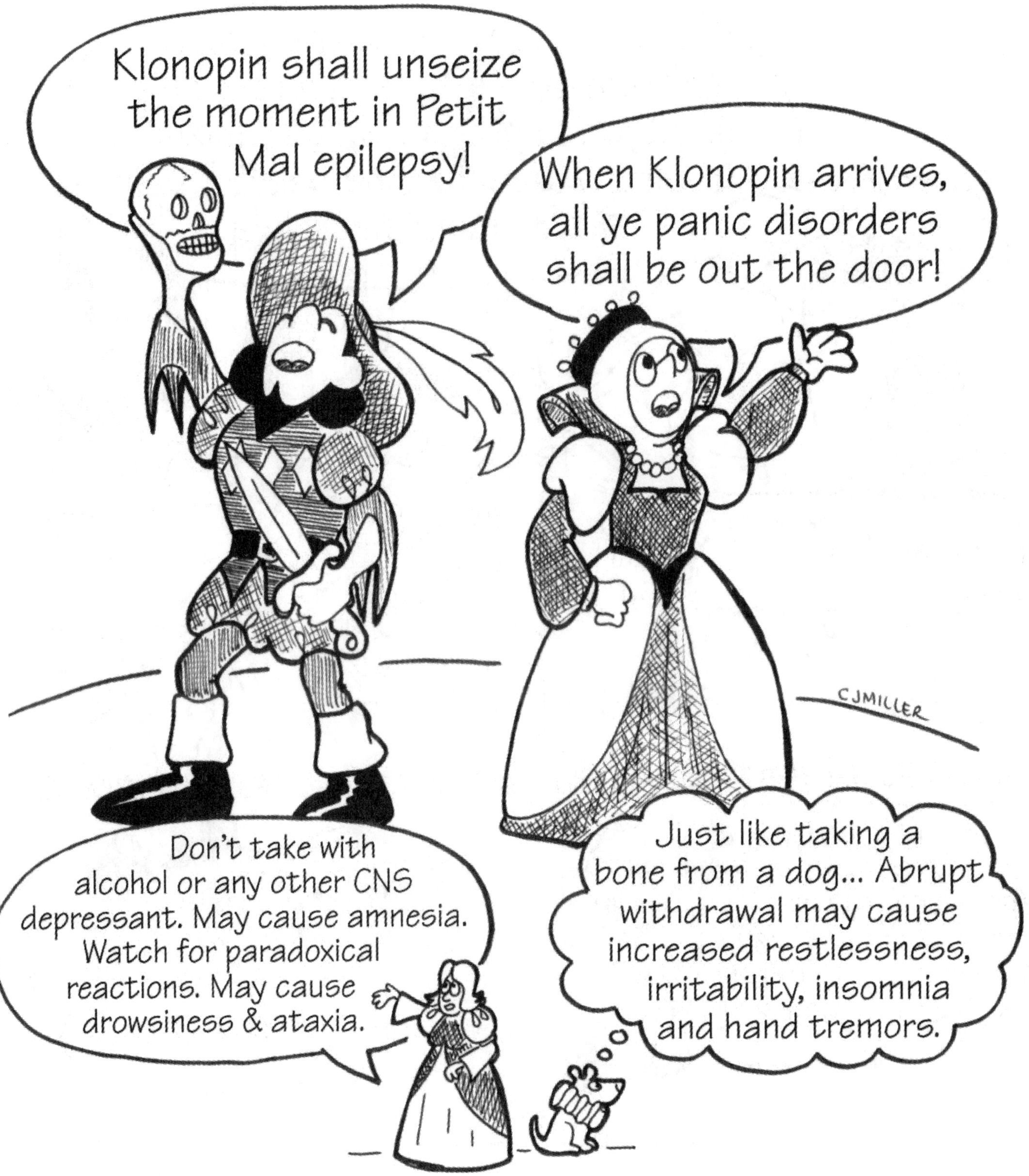
Klonopin shall unseize the moment in Petit Mal epilepsy!
When Klonopin arrives, all ye panic disorders shall be out the door!
CJMILLER
Don't take with alcohol or any other CNS depressant. May cause amnesia. Watch for paradoxical reactions. May cause drowsiness & ataxia.
Just like taking a bone from a dog... Abrupt withdrawal may cause increased restlessness, irritability, insomnia and hand tremors.

Gabapentin (Neurontin)

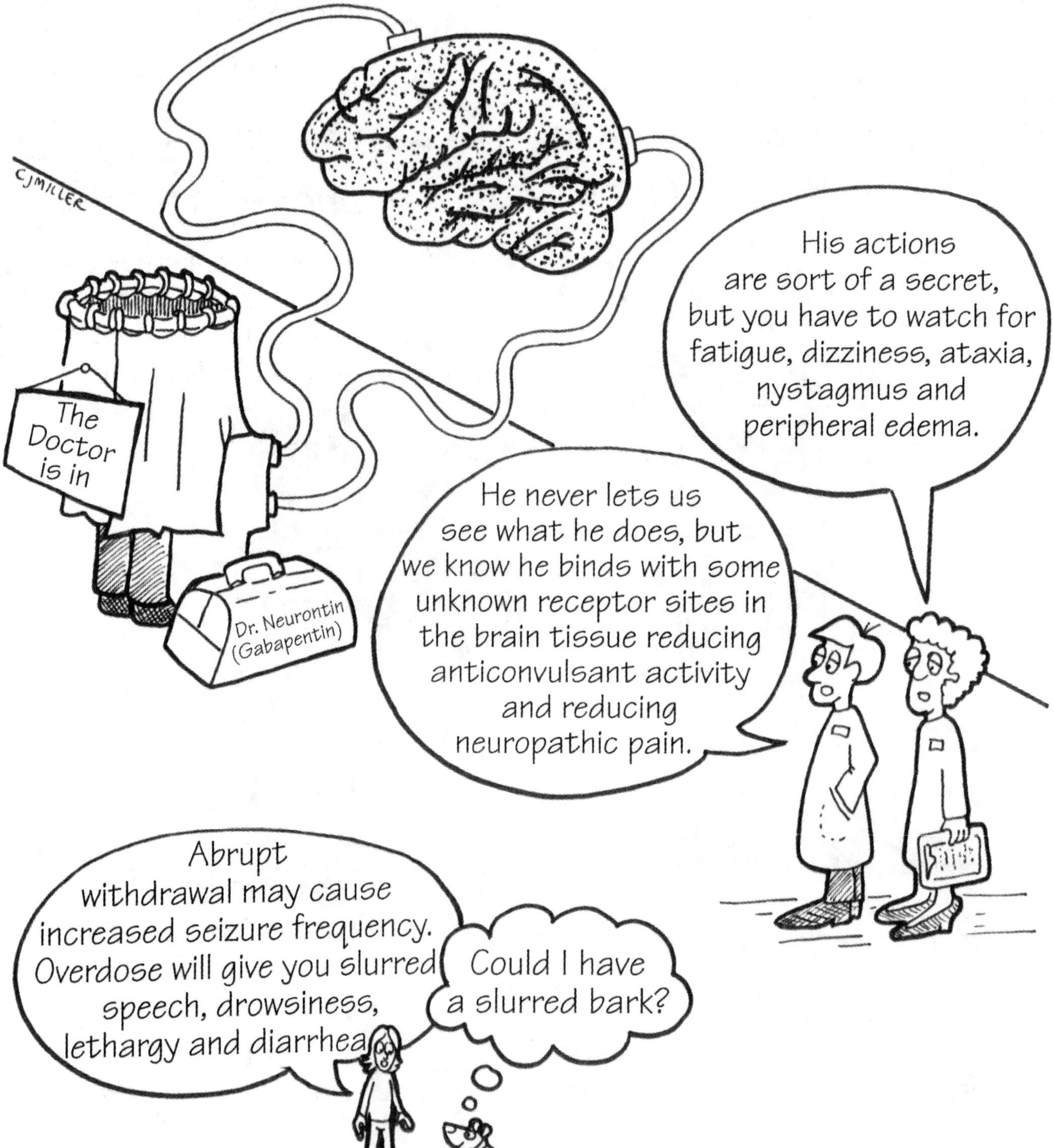
CJMILLER
The Doctor is in
Dr. Neurontin (Gabapentin)
His actions are sort of a secret, but you have to watch for fatigue, dizziness, ataxia, nystagmus and peripheral edema.
He never lets us see what he does, but we know he binds with some unknown receptor sites in the brain tissue reducing anticonvulsant activity and reducing neuropathic pain.
Abrupt withdrawal may cause increased seizure frequency. Overdose will give you slurred speech, drowsiness, lethargy and diarrhea.
Could I have a slurred bark?

Timolol (Timoptic)

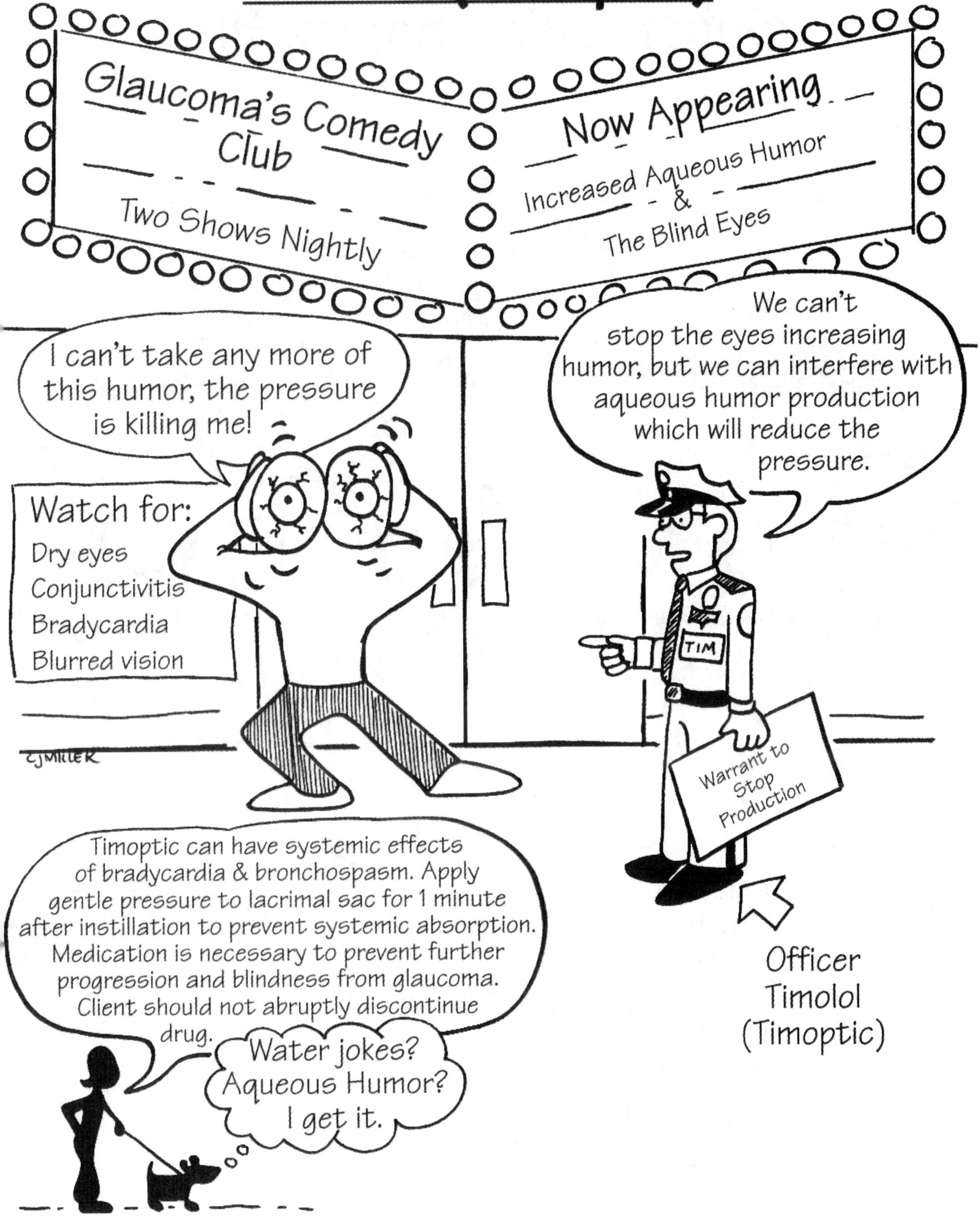
Glaucoma's Comedy Club
Two Shows Nightly
Now Appearing
Increased Aqueous Humor & The Blind Eyes
I can't take any more of this humor, the pressure is killing me!
We can't stop the eyes increasing humor, but we can interfere with aqueous humor production which will reduce the pressure.
Watch for:
Dry eyes
Conjunctivitis
Bradycardia
Blurred vision
TIM
Warrant to Stop Production
CJMILLER
Timoptic can have systemic effects of bradycardia & bronchospasm. Apply gentle pressure to lacrimal sac for 1 minute after instillation to prevent systemic absorption. Medication is necessary to prevent further progression and blindness from glaucoma. Client should not abruptly discontinue drug.
Water jokes? Aqueous Humor? I get it.
Officer Timolol (Timoptic)

Topical Vasoconstrictors

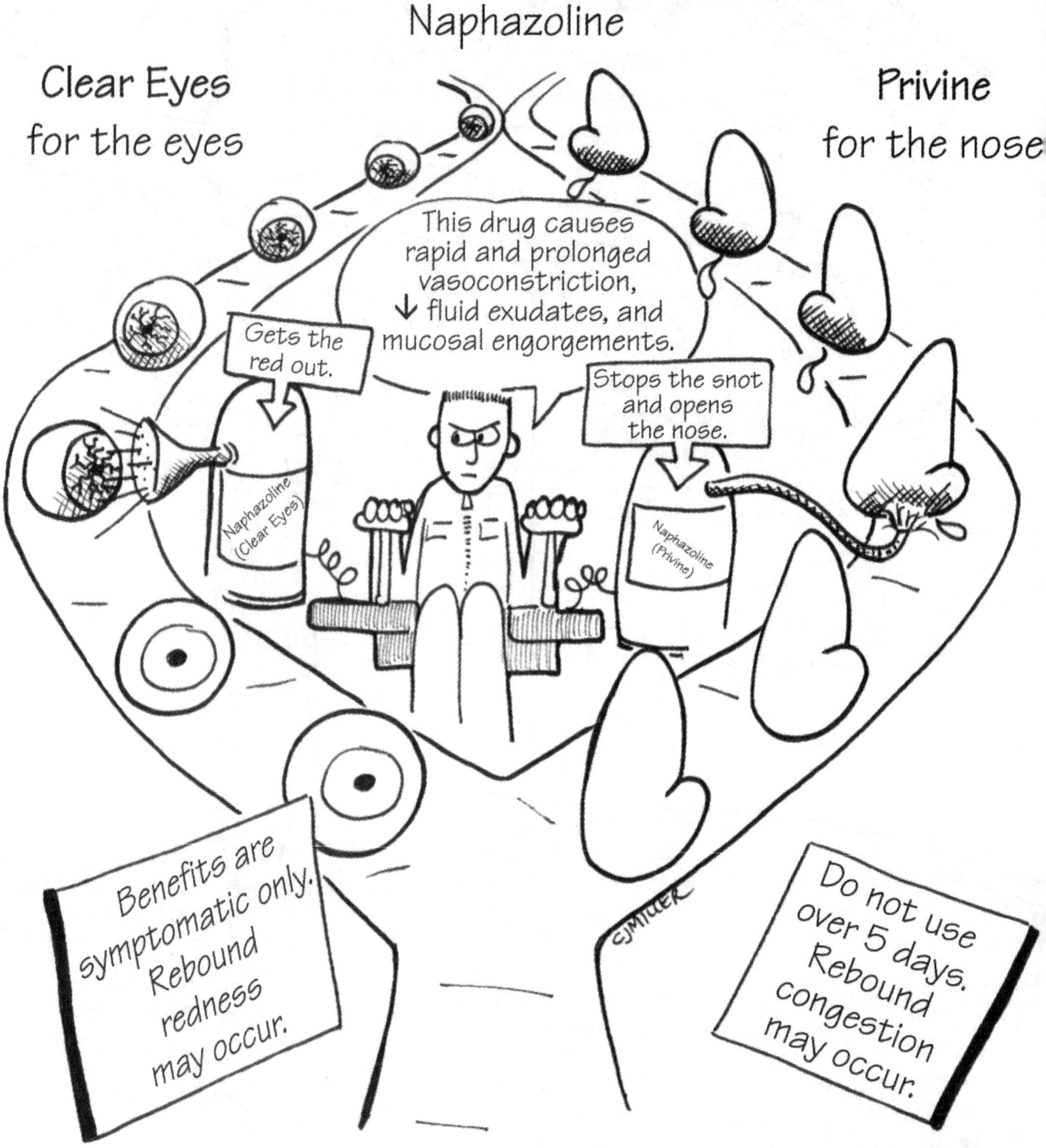
Naphazoline
Clear Eyes
for the eyes
Privine
for the nose
This drug causes rapid and prolonged vasoconstriction, ↓ fluid exudates, and mucosal engorgements.
Gets the red out.
Stops the snot and opens the nose.
Naphazoline (Clear Eyes)
Naphazoline (Privine)
Benefits are symptomatic only. Rebound redness may occur.
Do not use over 5 days. Rebound congestion may occur.
CJMILLER

Antigout

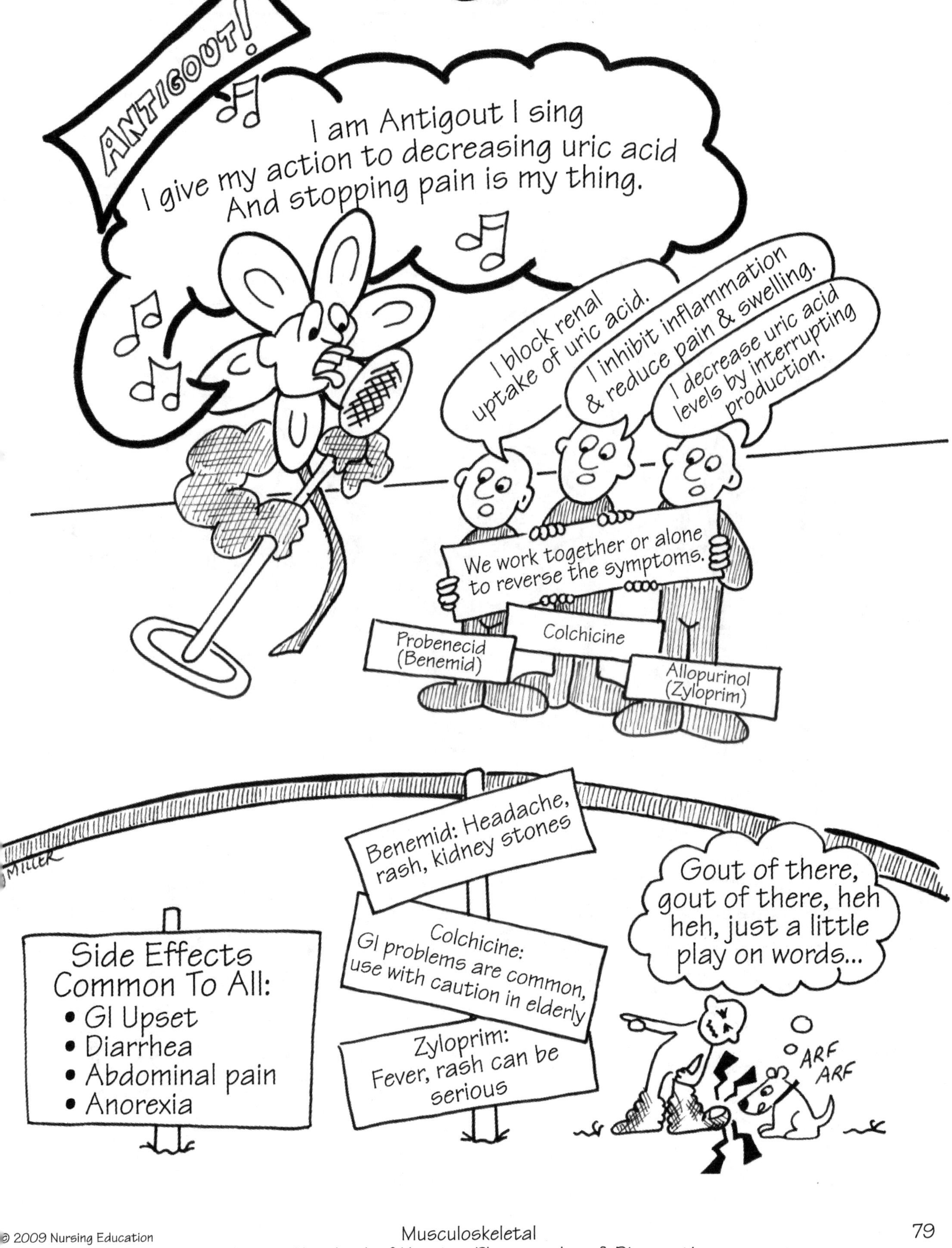
ANTIGOUT!
I am Antigout I sing
I give my action to decreasing uric acid
And stopping pain is my thing.
I block renal uptake of uric acid.
I inhibit inflammation & reduce pain & swelling.
I decrease uric acid levels by interrupting production.
We work together or alone to reverse the symptoms.
Probenecid (Benemid)
Colchicine
Allopurinol (Zyloprim)
MILLER
Benemid: Headache, rash, kidney stones
Colchicine: GI problems are common, use with caution in elderly
Zyloprim: Fever, rash can be serious
Side Effects Common To All:
• GI Upset
• Diarrhea
• Abdominal pain
• Anorexia
Gout of there, gout of there, heh heh, just a little play on words...
ARF ARF

Biophosphonate Therapy

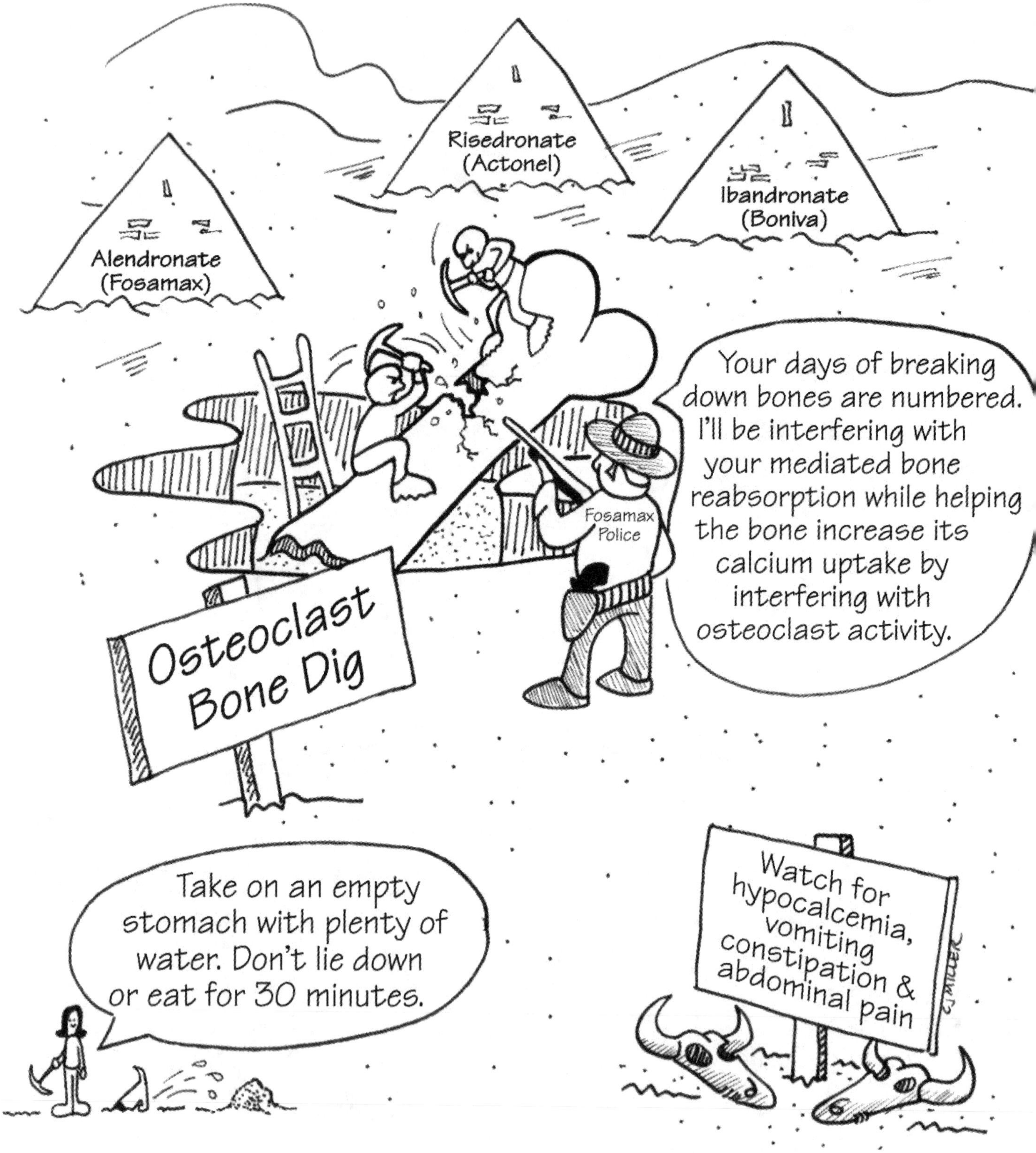
Risedronate
(Actonel)
Ibandronate
(Boniva)
Alendronate
(Fosamax)
Your days of breaking down bones are numbered. I'll be interfering with your mediated bone reabsorption while helping the bone increase its calcium uptake by interfering with osteoclast activity.
Fosamax Police
Osteoclast Bone Dig
Take on an empty stomach with plenty of water. Don't lie down or eat for 30 minutes.
Watch for hypocalcemia, vomiting constipation & abdominal pain
CJ MILLER

Calcitonin-Salmon (Calcimar)

"When diet alone just isn't enough...
Calcimar, a bone resorption inhibitor."

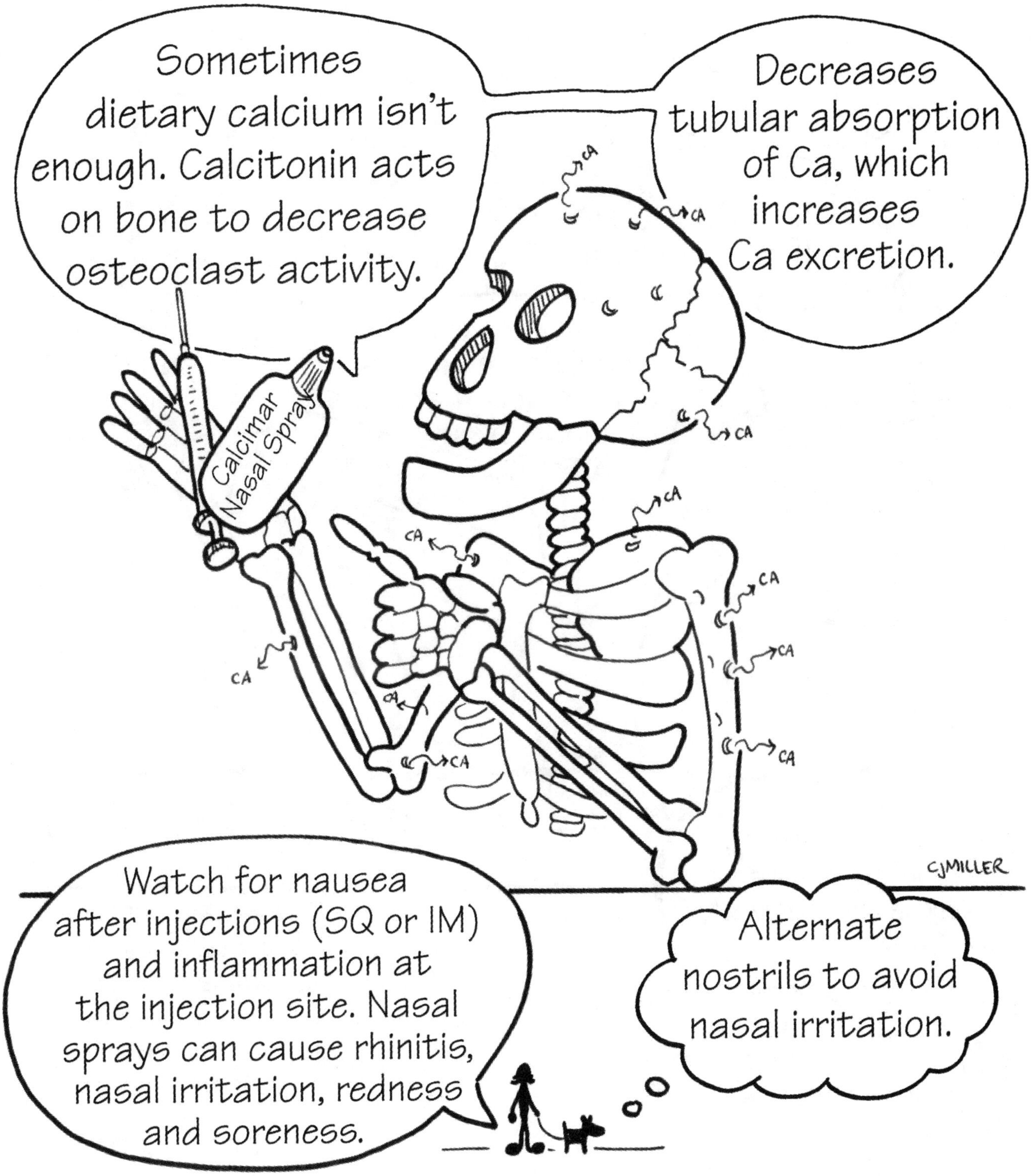

Sometimes dietary calcium isn't enough. Calcitonin acts on bone to decrease osteoclast activity.
Decreases tubular absorption of Ca, which increases Ca excretion.
Calcimar Nasal Spray
CA
CJMILLER
Watch for nausea after injections (SQ or IM) and inflammation at the injection site. Nasal sprays can cause rhinitis, nasal irritation, redness and soreness.
Alternate nostrils to avoid nasal irritation.

Calcium Supplements (Oral)

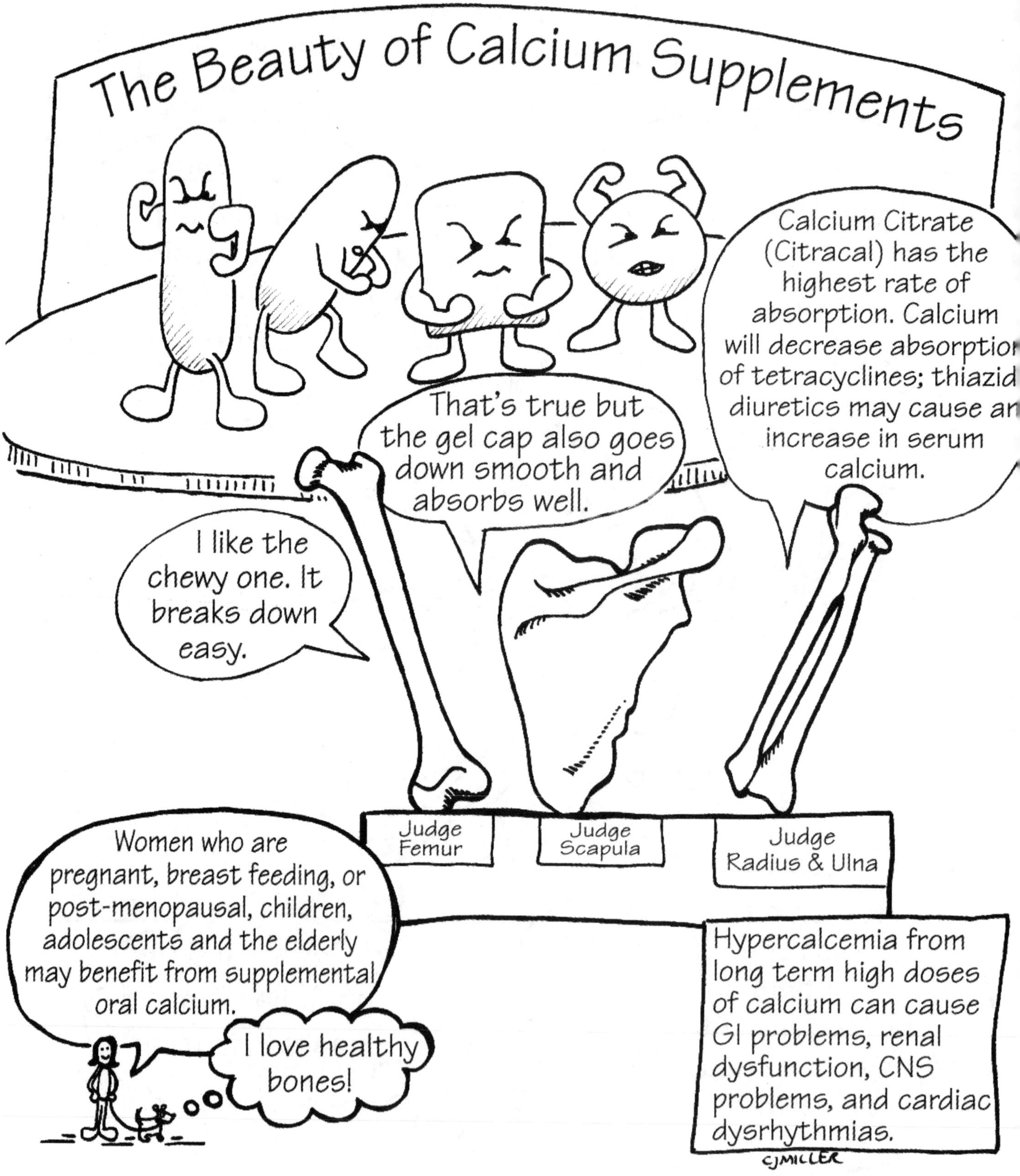

The Beauty of Calcium Supplements
Calcium Citrate (Citracal) has the highest rate of absorption. Calcium will decrease absorptio of tetracyclines; thiazid diuretics may cause an increase in serum calcium.
That's true but the gel cap also goes down smooth and absorbs well.
I like the chewy one. It breaks down easy.
Judge Femur
Judge Scapula
Judge Radius & Ulna
Women who are pregnant, breast feeding, or post-menopausal, children, adolescents and the elderly may benefit from supplemental oral calcium.
I love healthy bones!
Hypercalcemia from long term high doses of calcium can cause GI problems, renal dysfunction, CNS problems, and cardiac dysrhythmias.
CJMILLER

Colecoxib (Celebrex)

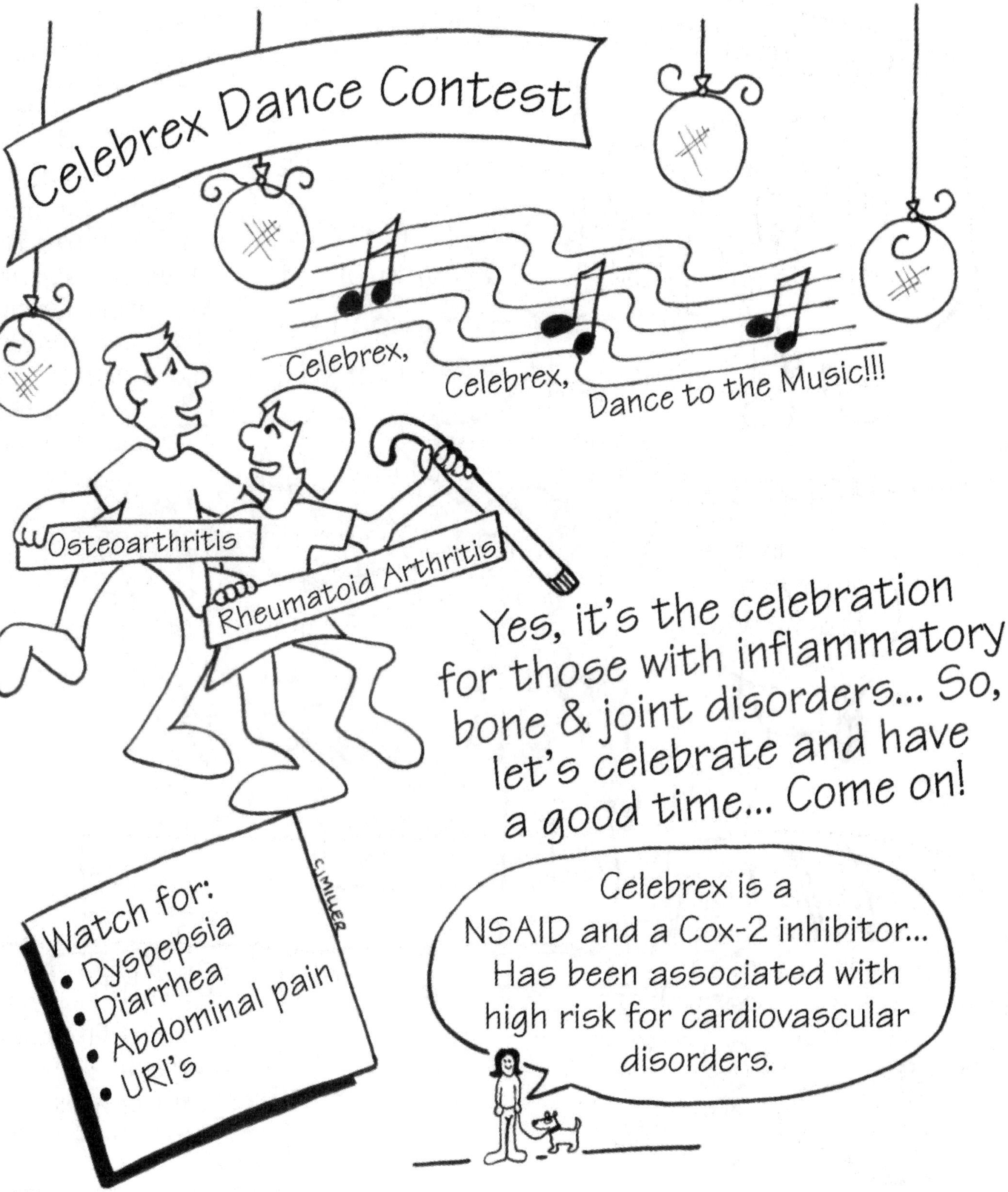

Celebrex Dance Contest
Celebrex,
Celebrex,
Dance to the Music!!!
Osteoarthritis
Rheumatoid Arthritis
Yes, it's the celebration for those with inflammatory bone & joint disorders... So, let's celebrate and have a good time... Come on!
Watch for:
• Dyspepsia
• Diarrhea
• Abdominal pain
• URI's
C. MILLER
Celebrex is a NSAID and a Cox-2 inhibitor... Has been associated with high risk for cardiovascular disorders.

Etodolac (Lodine)

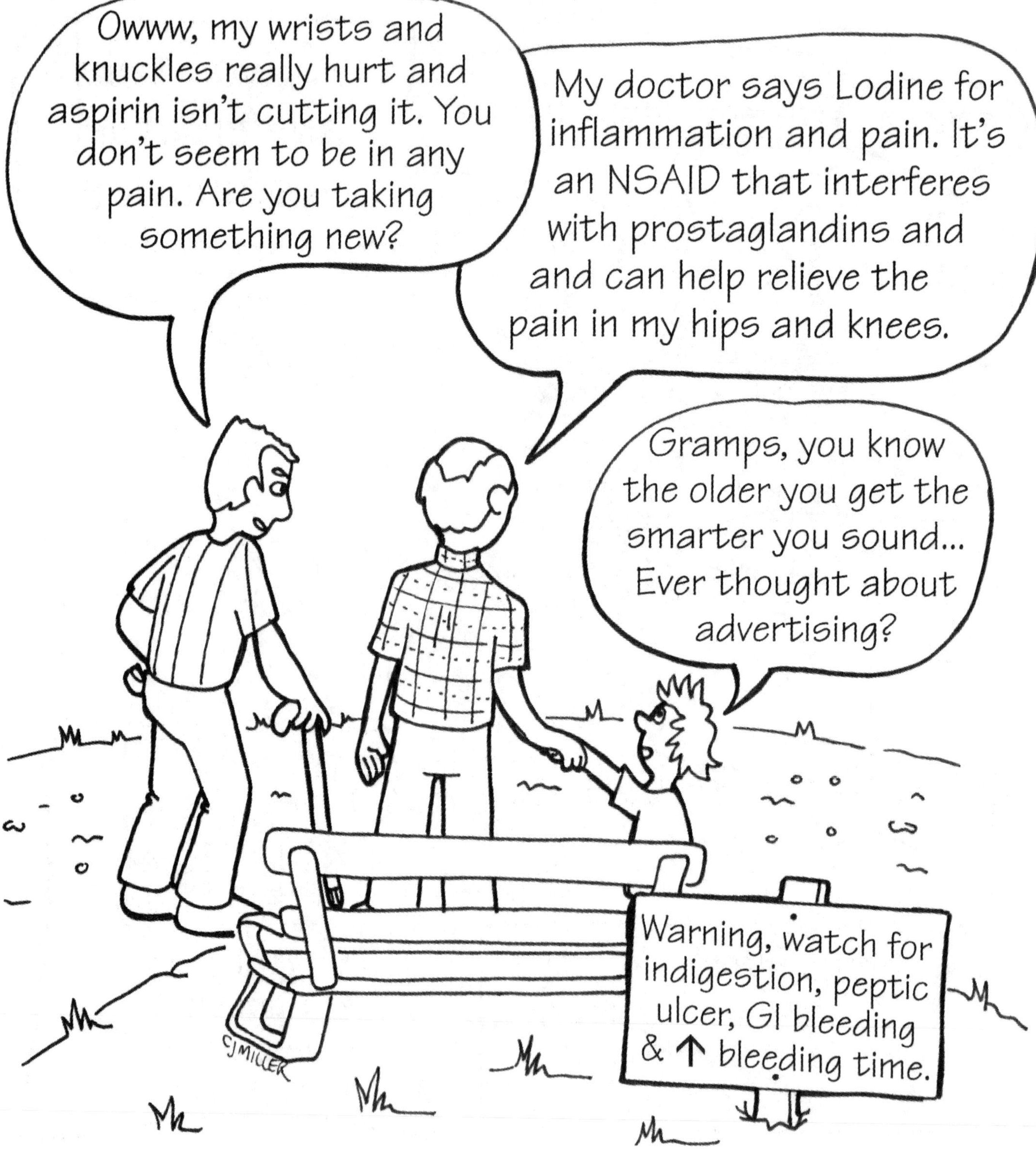

Owww, my wrists and knuckles really hurt and aspirin isn't cutting it. You don't seem to be in any pain. Are you taking something new?
My doctor says Lodine for inflammation and pain. It's an NSAID that interferes with prostaglandins and and can help relieve the pain in my hips and knees.
Gramps, you know the older you get the smarter you sound... Ever thought about advertising?
Warning, watch for indigestion, peptic ulcer, GI bleeding & ↑ bleeding time.
CJ MILLER

Erectile Dysfunction Drugs

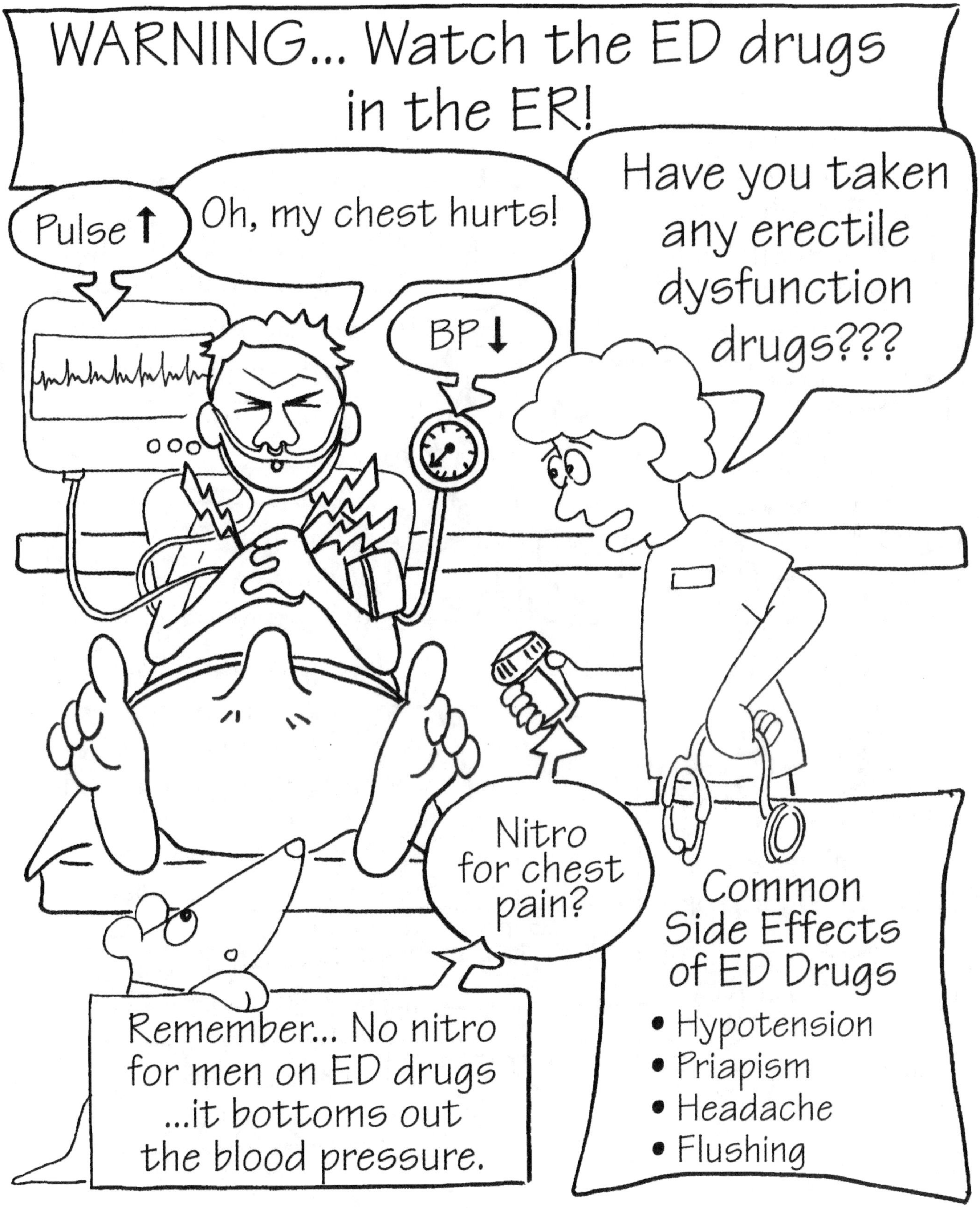
WARNING... Watch the ED drugs in the ER!
Pulse ↑
Oh, my chest hurts!
Have you taken any erectile dysfunction drugs???
BP ↓
Nitro for chest pain?
Remember... No nitro for men on ED drugs ...it bottoms out the blood pressure.
Common Side Effects of ED Drugs
• Hypotension
• Priapism
• Headache
• Flushing

Medroxyprogesterone (Depo Provera)

"It's Not Just For Birth Control"

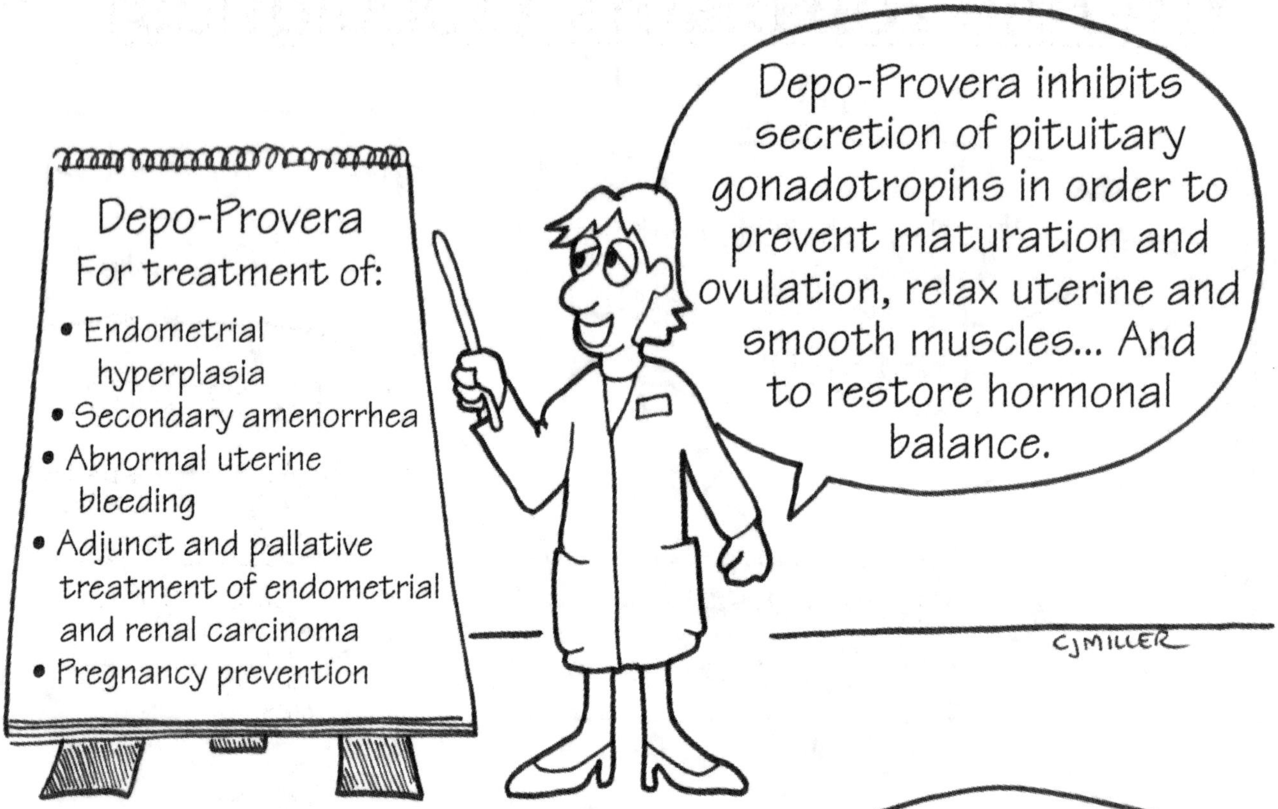
Depo-Provera
For treatment of:
• Endometrial hyperplasia
• Secondary amenorrhea
• Abnormal uterine bleeding
• Adjunct and pallative treatment of endometrial and renal carcinoma
• Pregnancy prevention
Depo-Provera inhibits secretion of pituitary gonadotropins in order to prevent maturation and ovulation, relax uterine and smooth muscles... And to restore hormonal balance.
CJMILLER

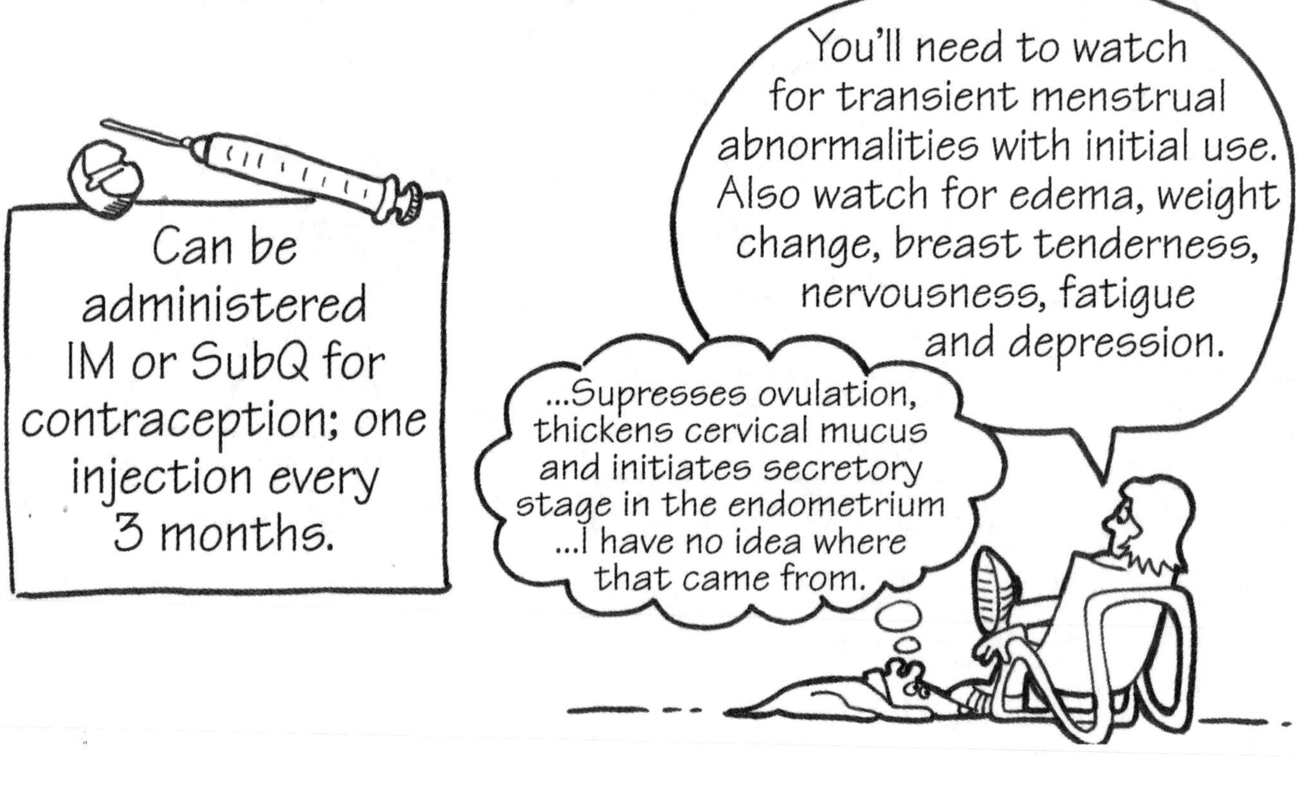
Can be administered IM or SubQ for contraception; one injection every 3 months.
You'll need to watch for transient menstrual abnormalities with initial use. Also watch for edema, weight change, breast tenderness, nervousness, fatigue and depression.
...Supresses ovulation, thickens cervical mucus and initiates secretory stage in the endometrium ...I have no idea where that came from.

Uterine Relaxants (Tocolytics)

I. Indomethacin
(NSAID)

N. Nifedipine
(CA Channel Blocker)

M. Magnesium Sulfate

T. Terbutaline
(Adrenergic Agonist)

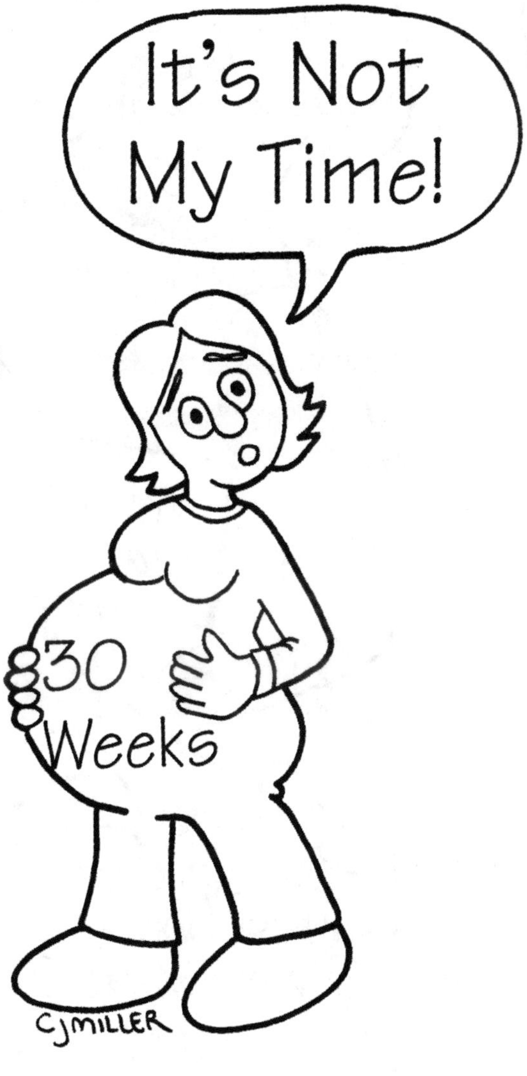
It's Not My Time!
30 Weeks
CJMILLER

RhoGAM

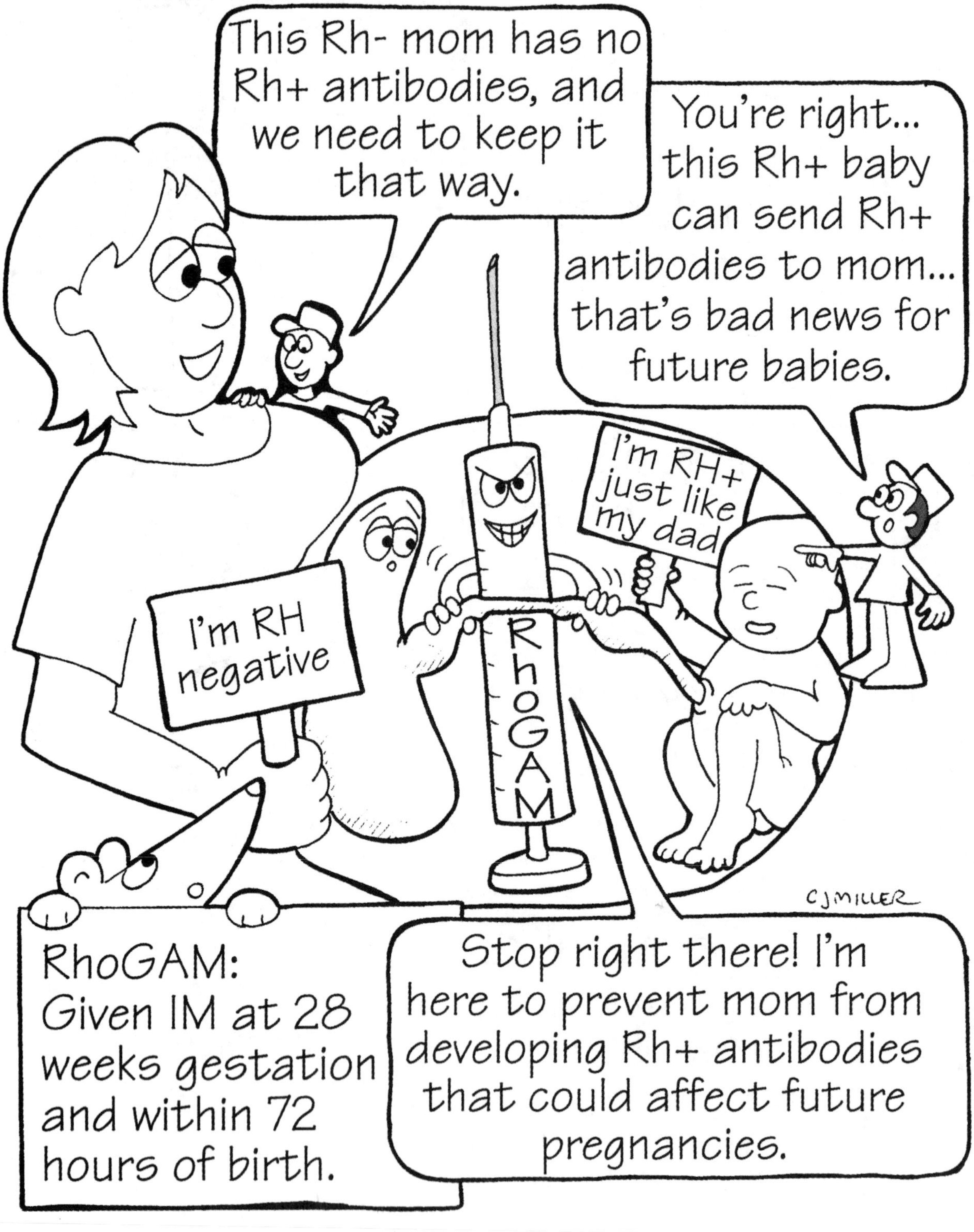

This Rh- mom has no Rh+ antibodies, and we need to keep it that way.
You're right... this Rh+ baby can send Rh+ antibodies to mom... that's bad news for future babies.
I'm RH+ just like my dad
I'm RH negative
RhoGAM
CJMILLER
RhoGAM: Given IM at 28 weeks gestation and within 72 hours of birth.
Stop right there! I'm here to prevent mom from developing Rh+ antibodies that could affect future pregnancies.

Oxytocin (Pitocin)

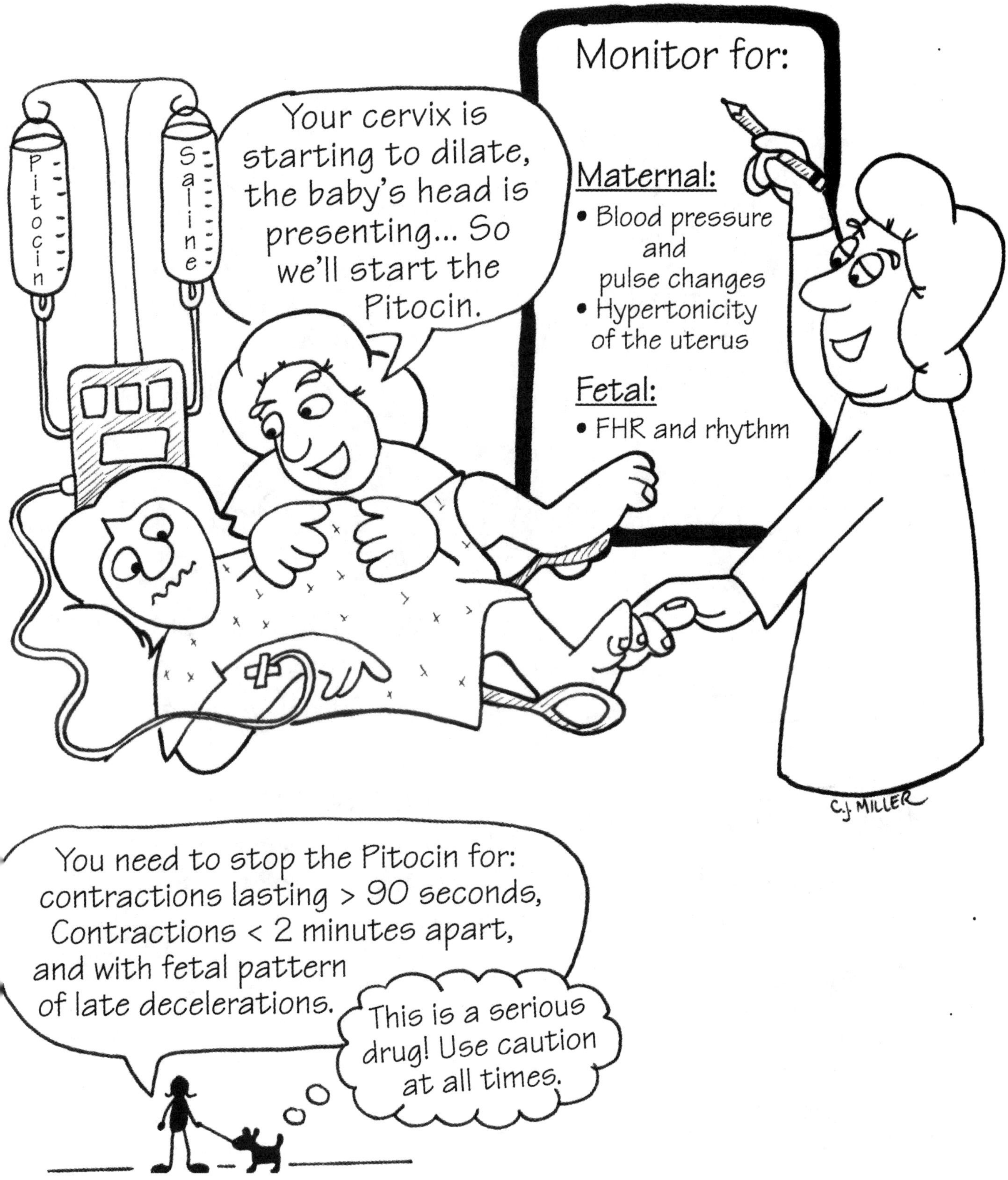
Pitocin
Saline
Your cervix is starting to dilate, the baby's head is presenting... So we'll start the Pitocin.
Monitor for:
Maternal:
• Blood pressure and pulse changes
• Hypertonicity of the uterus
Fetal:
• FHR and rhythm
C.J. MILLER
You need to stop the Pitocin for: contractions lasting > 90 seconds, Contractions < 2 minutes apart, and with fetal pattern of late decelerations.
This is a serious drug! Use caution at all times.

Tolterodine (Detrol)

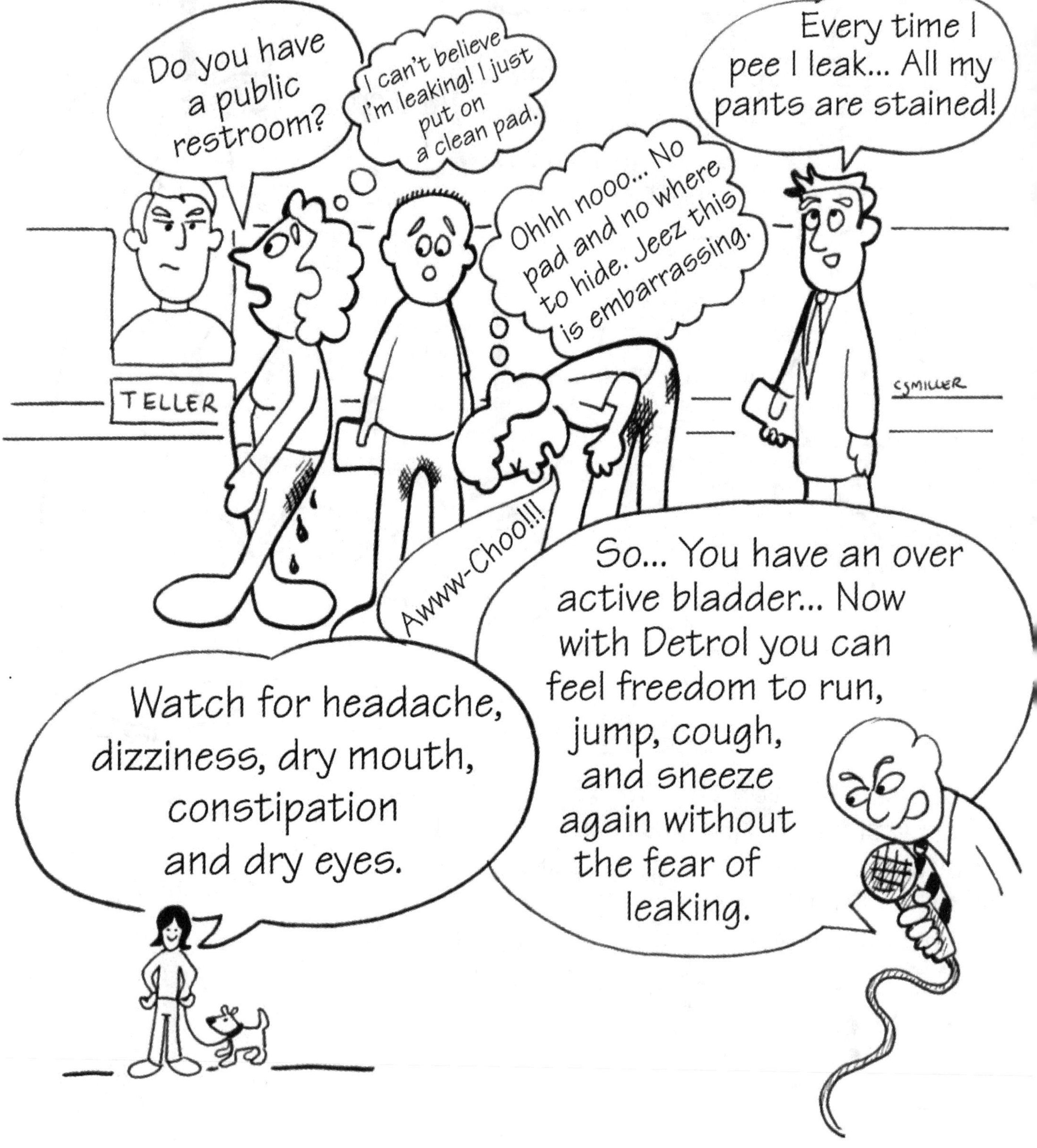
Do you have a public restroom?
I can't believe I'm leaking! I just put on a clean pad.
Every time I pee I leak... All my pants are stained!
Ohhh nooo... No pad and no where to hide. Jeez this is embarrassing.
TELLER
CSMILLER
Awww-Choo!!!
So... You have an over active bladder... Now with Detrol you can feel freedom to run, jump, cough, and sneeze again without the fear of leaking.
Watch for headache, dizziness, dry mouth, constipation and dry eyes.

Azathioprine (Imuran)

"Suppressing the Body's Defenses"

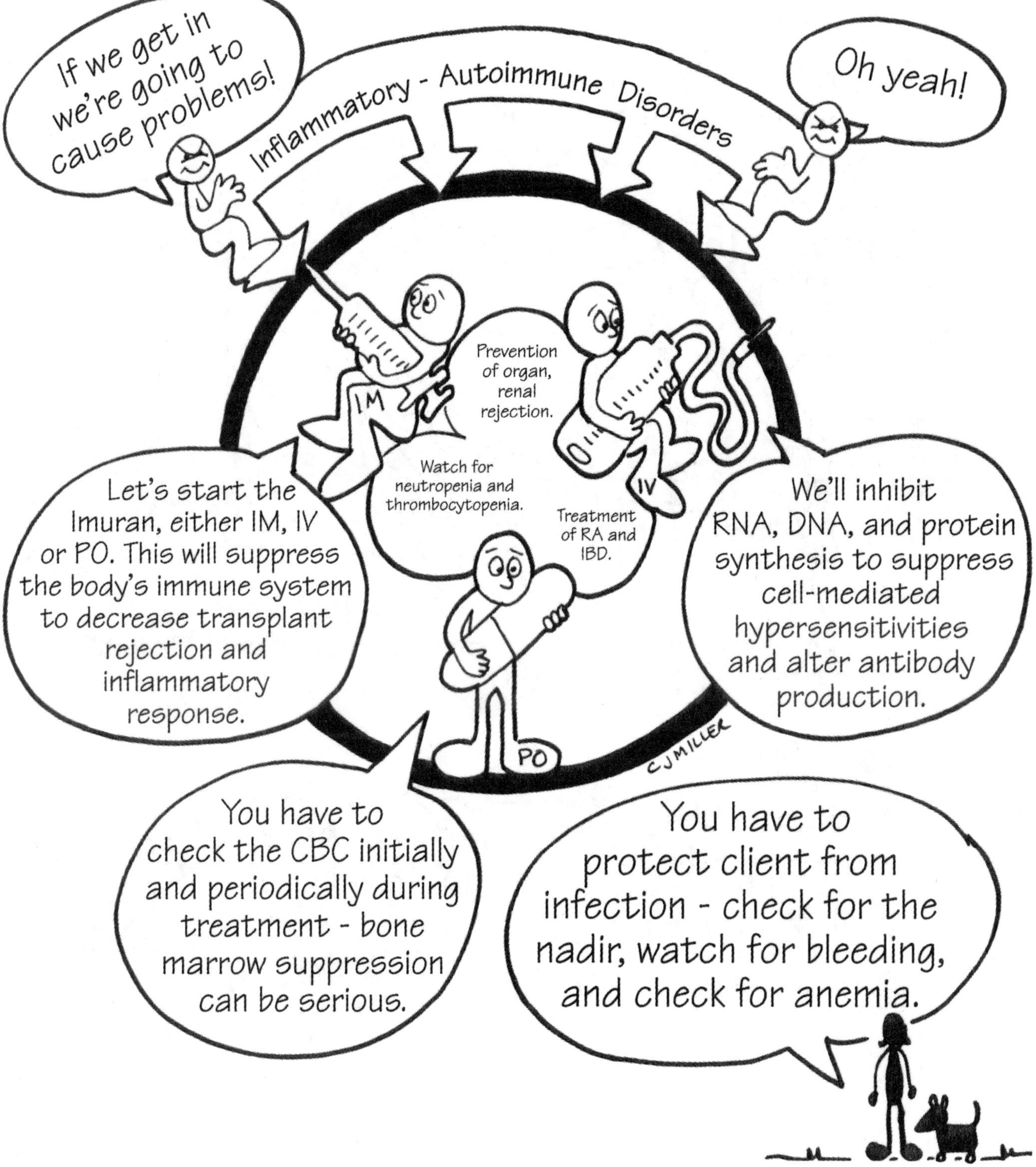

If we get in we're going to cause problems!
Oh yeah!
Inflammatory - Autoimmune Disorders
IM
IV
PO
Prevention of organ, renal rejection.
Watch for neutropenia and thrombocytopenia.
Treatment of RA and IBD.
Let's start the Imuran, either IM, IV or PO. This will suppress the body's immune system to decrease transplant rejection and inflammatory response.
We'll inhibit RNA, DNA, and protein synthesis to suppress cell-mediated hypersensitivities and alter antibody production.
You have to check the CBC initially and periodically during treatment - bone marrow suppression can be serious.
You have to protect client from infection - check for the nadir, watch for bleeding, and check for anemia.
CJMILLER

Drug Interactions & Grapefruit

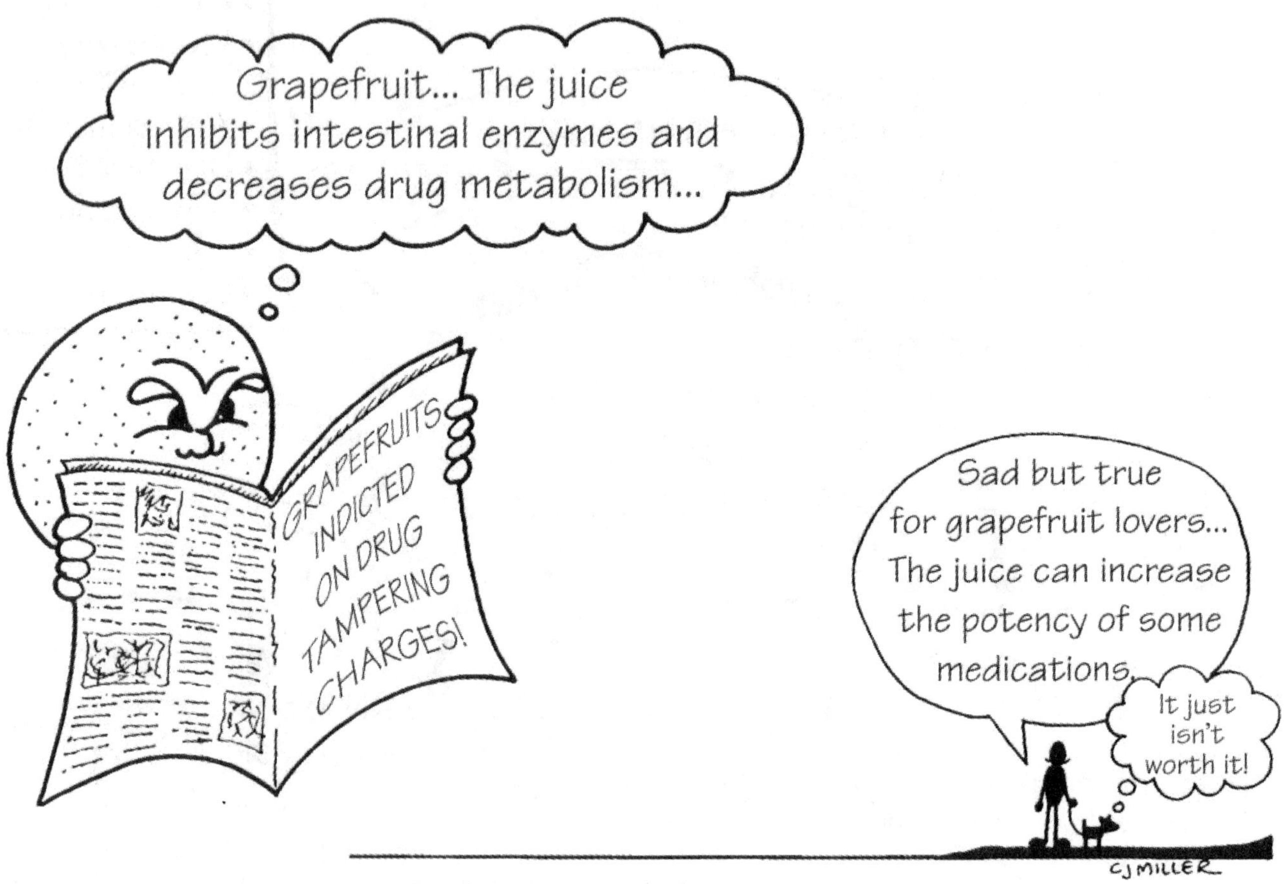
Grapefruit... The juice inhibits intestinal enzymes and decreases drug metabolism...
GRAPEFRUITS INDICTED ON DRUG TAMPERING CHARGES!
Sad but true for grapefruit lovers... The juice can increase the potency of some medications.
It just isn't worth it!
CJMILLER

DON'T USE WITH US...

Felodipine (Plendil)
Nifedipine (Procardia)
Amolodipine (Norvasc)
Verapamil (Calan)
Carbamazepine (Tegretol)
Buspirone (Buspar)
Lovastatin (Mevacor)
Calcium Channel Blockers
Other Drugs

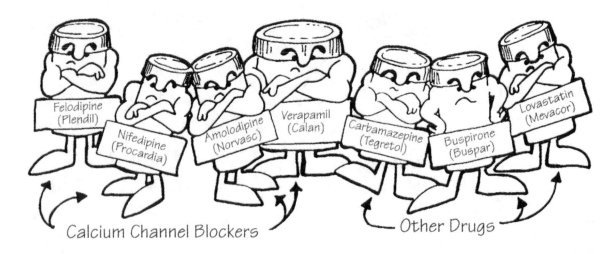

Midazolam (Versed)

Moments Not Remembered

Watch for:

- Respiratory depression
- Arrhythmias
- Hypotension
- Unresponsiveness
- Agitation
- Confusion

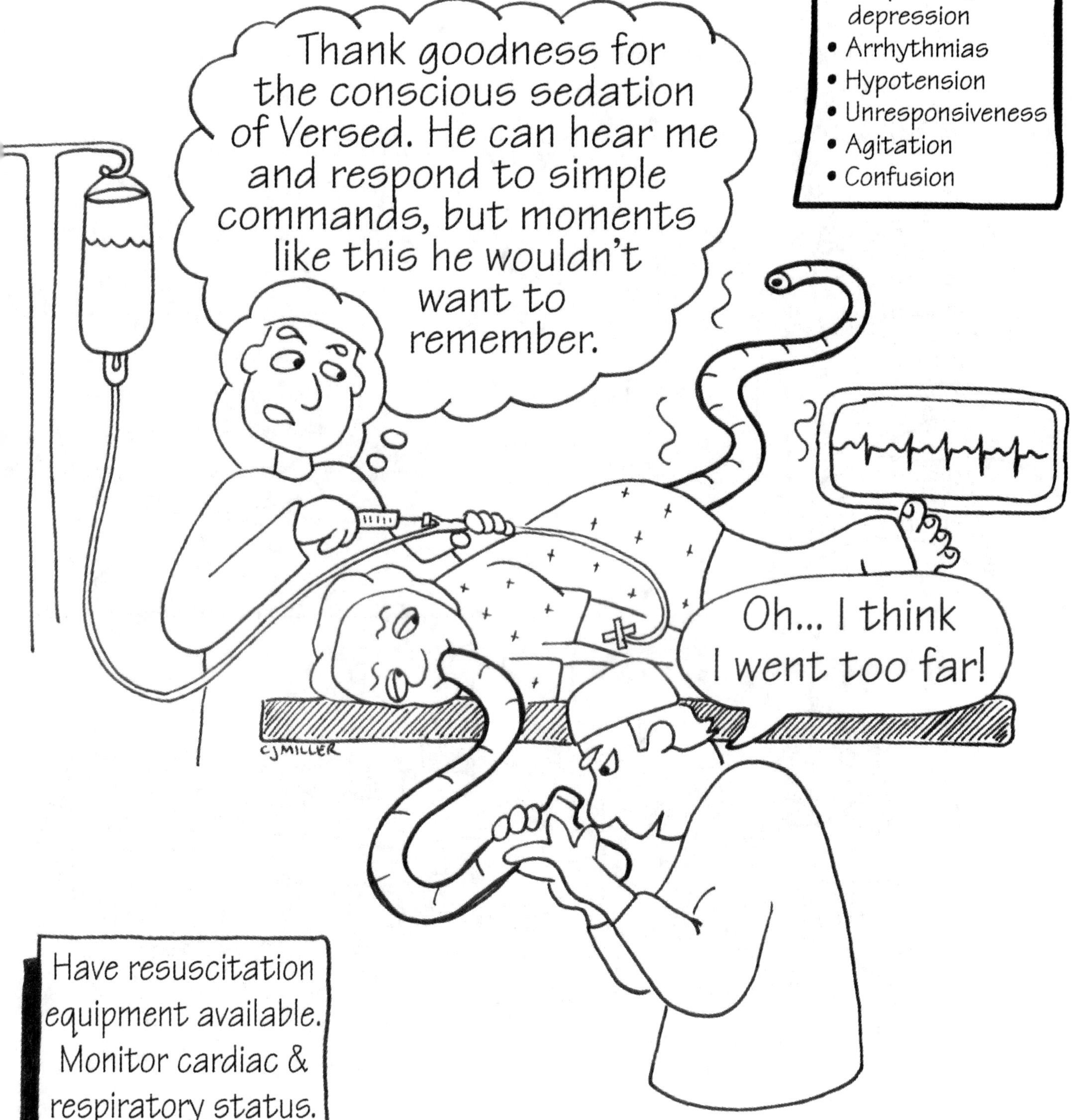
Thank goodness for the conscious sedation of Versed. He can hear me and respond to simple commands, but moments like this he wouldn't want to remember.
Oh... I think I went too far!
CJMILLER

Have resuscitation equipment available. Monitor cardiac & respiratory status.

Phenazopyridine (Pyridium)

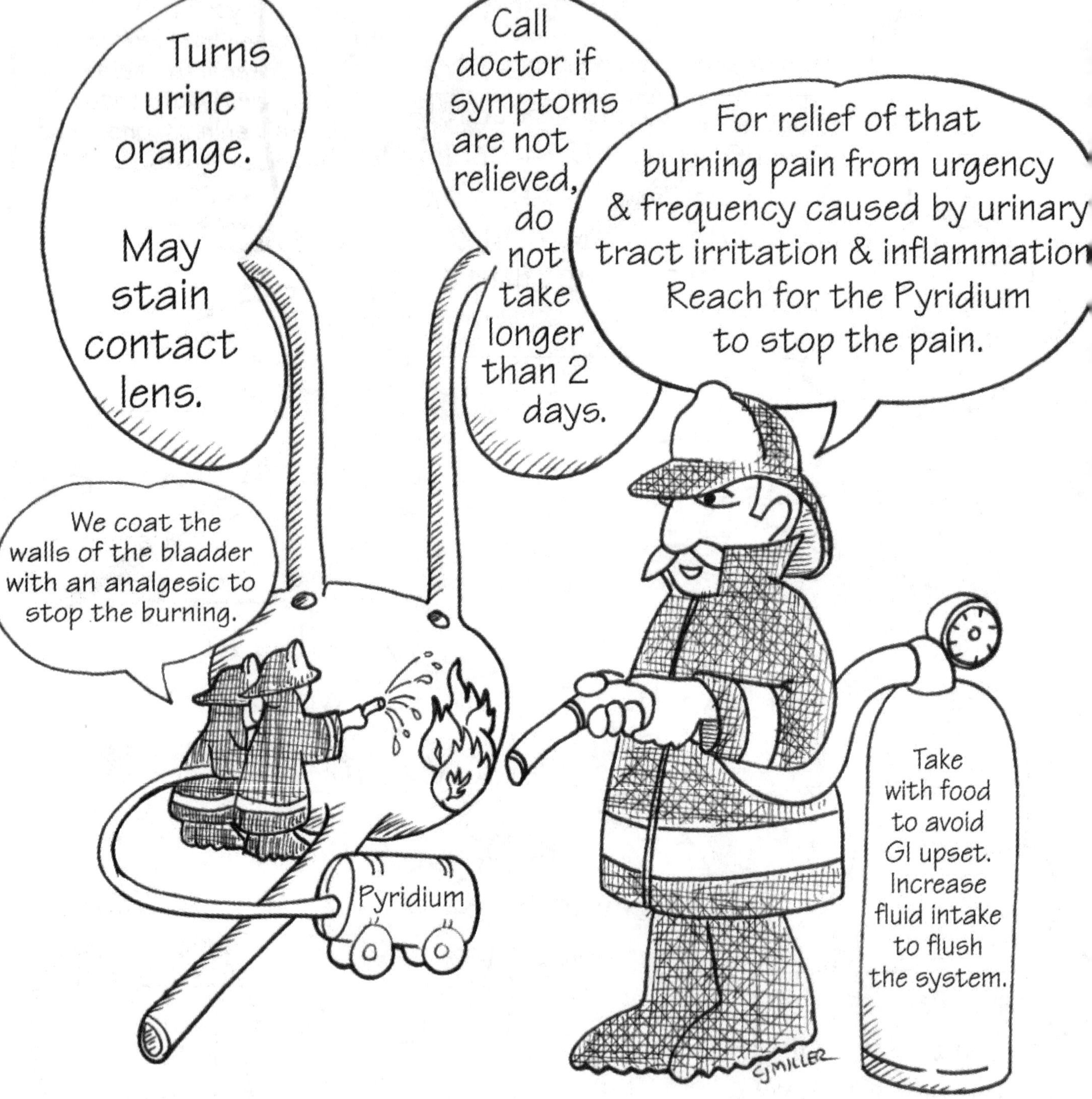

Turns urine orange.
May stain contact lens.
Call doctor if symptoms are not relieved, do not take longer than 2 days.
For relief of that burning pain from urgency & frequency caused by urinary tract irritation & inflammation Reach for the Pyridium to stop the pain.
We coat the walls of the bladder with an analgesic to stop the burning.
Pyridium
Take with food to avoid GI upset. Increase fluid intake to flush the system.
G MILLER

Potassium Chloride (IV & PO)

Life Hangs in the Balance

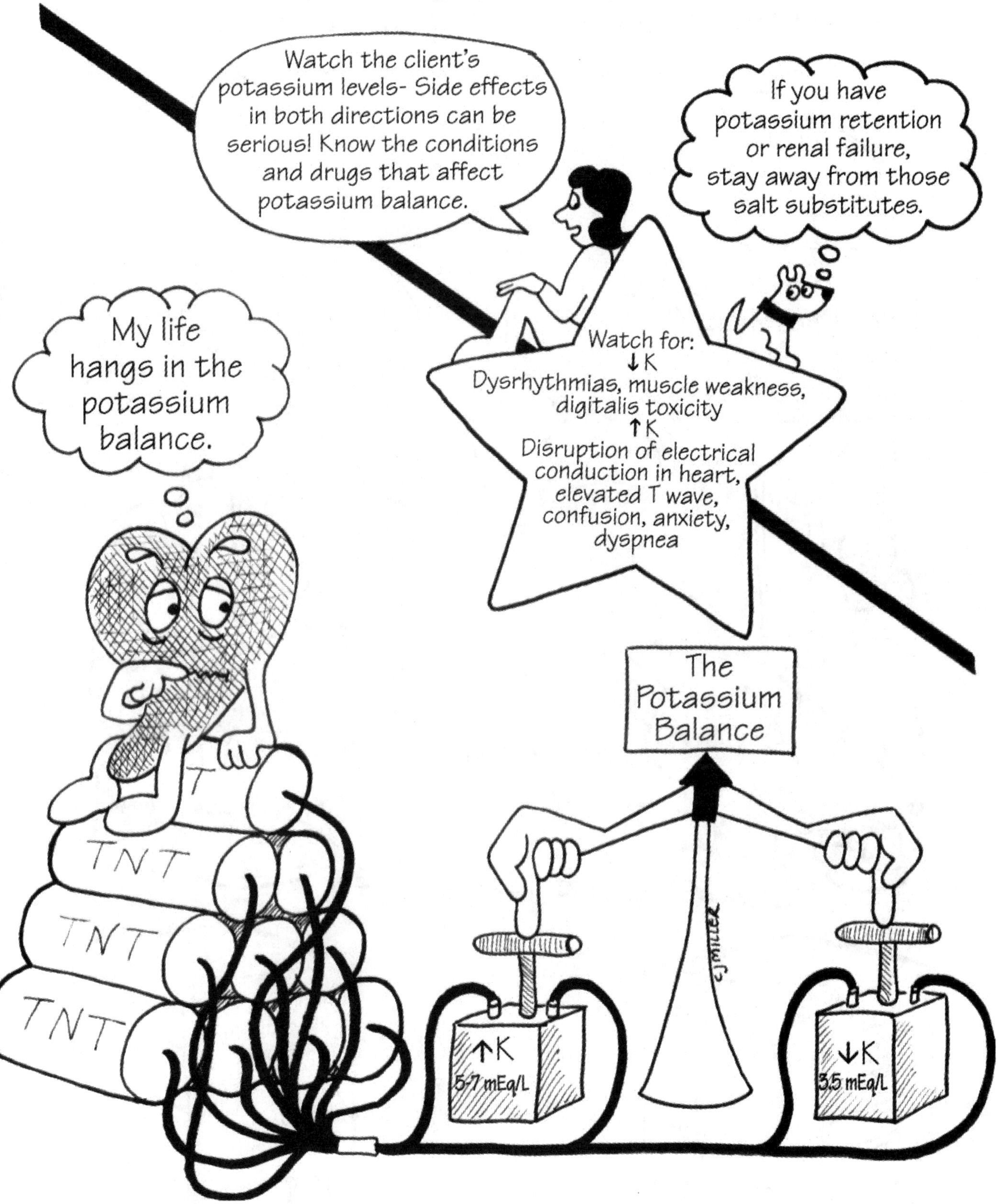

Watch the client's potassium levels- Side effects in both directions can be serious! Know the conditions and drugs that affect potassium balance.
If you have potassium retention or renal failure, stay away from those salt substitutes.
My life hangs in the potassium balance.
Watch for:
↓K
Dysrhythmias, muscle weakness, digitalis toxicity
↑K
Disruption of electrical conduction in heart, elevated T wave, confusion, anxiety, dyspnea
The Potassium Balance
TNT
TNT
TNT
T
↑K
5-7 mEq/L
↓K
3.5 mEq/L
CJ MILLER

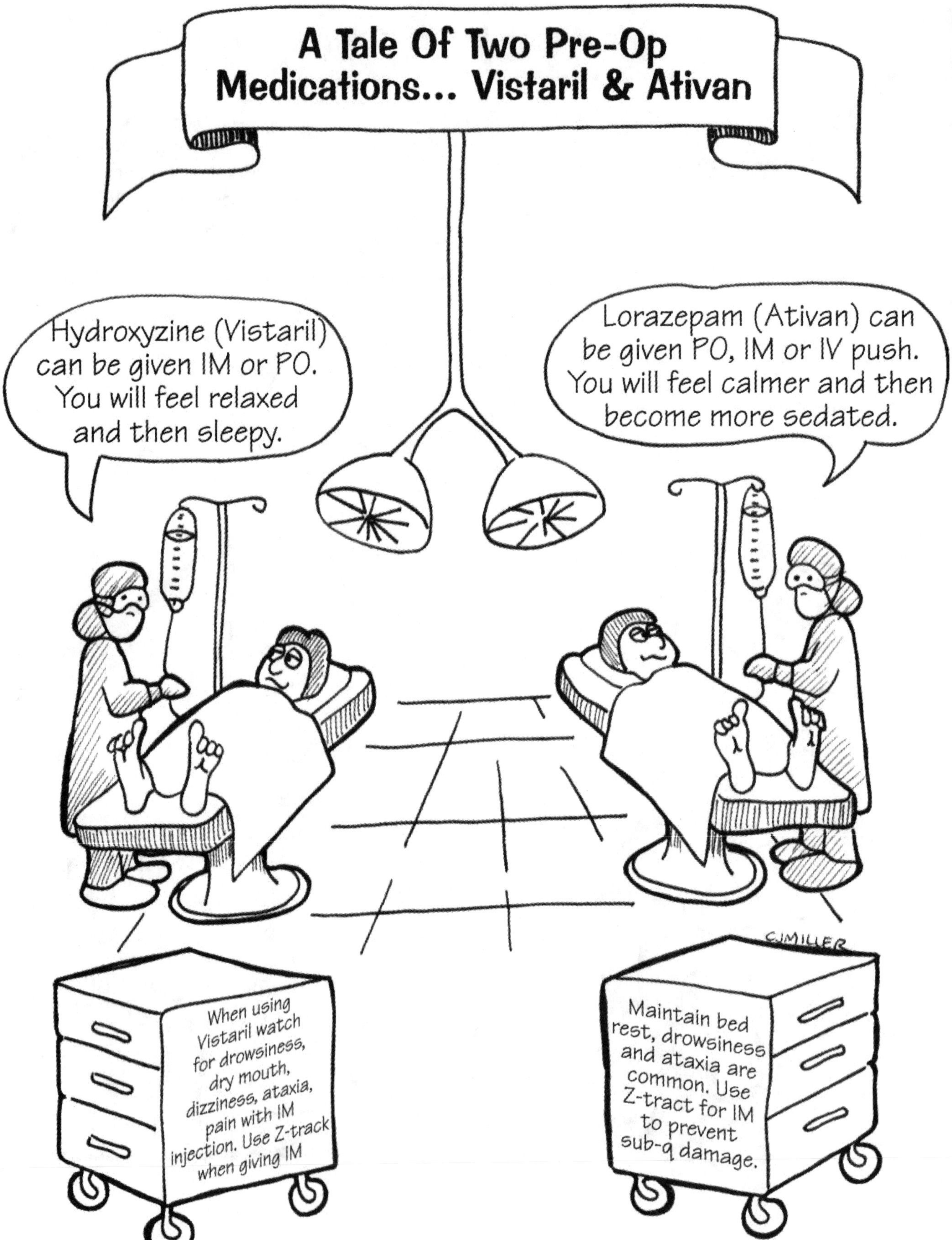
A Tale Of Two Pre-Op Medications... Vistaril & Ativan
Hydroxyzine (Vistaril) can be given IM or PO. You will feel relaxed and then sleepy.
Lorazepam (Ativan) can be given PO, IM or IV push. You will feel calmer and then become more sedated.
When using Vistaril watch for drowsiness, dry mouth, dizziness, ataxia, pain with IM injection. Use Z-track when giving IM
Maintain bed rest, drowsiness and ataxia are common. Use Z-tract for IM to prevent sub-q damage.
CJMILLER

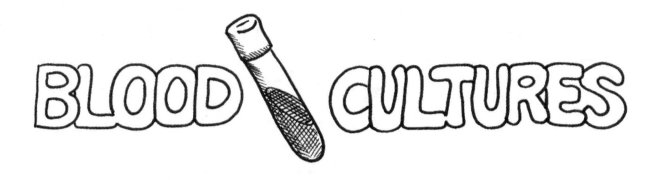

BLOOD CULTURES

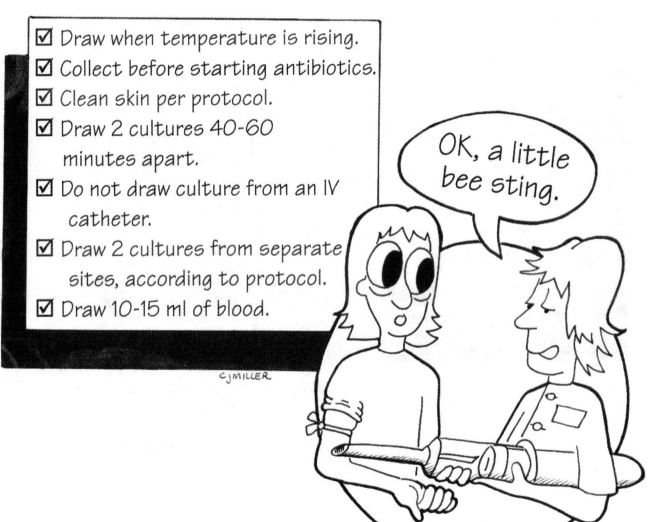

- ☑ Draw when temperature is rising.
- ☑ Collect before starting antibiotics.
- ☑ Clean skin per protocol.
- ☑ Draw 2 cultures 40-60 minutes apart.
- ☑ Do not draw culture from an IV catheter.
- ☑ Draw 2 cultures from separate sites, according to protocol.
- ☑ Draw 10-15 ml of blood.

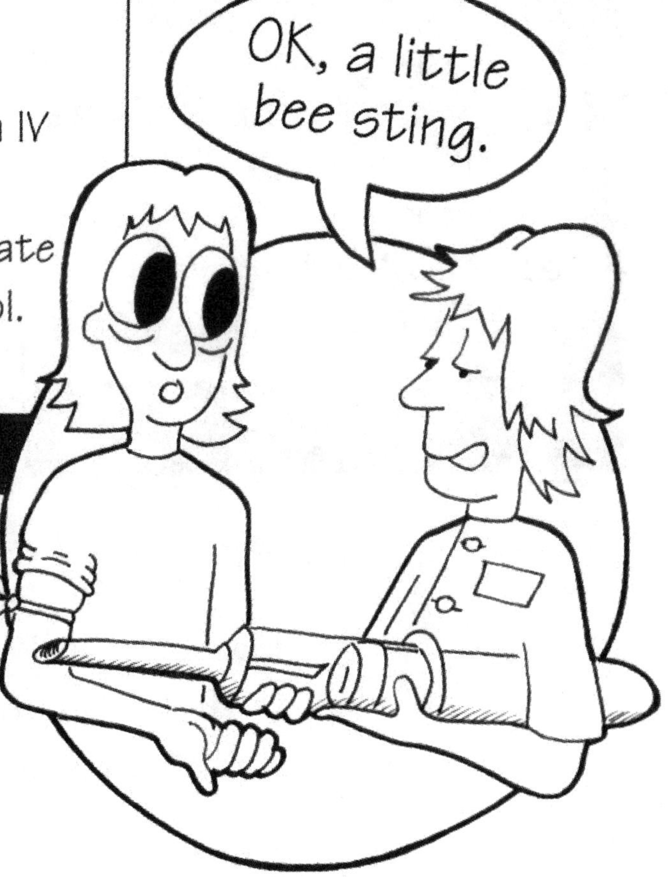
OK, a little bee sting.

CJMILLER

SPUTUM CULTURES

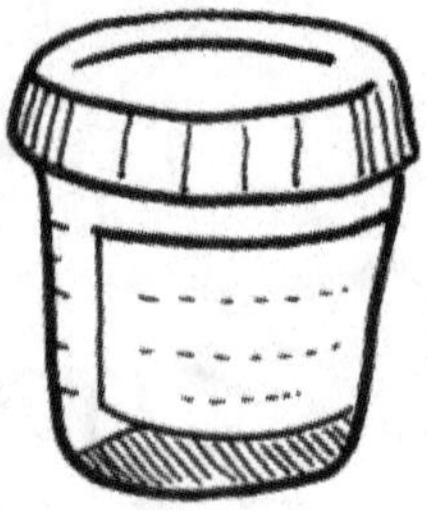

- ☑ Collect sample first thing in the morning for TB cultures.
- ☑ Collect ASAP for other sputum diagnostics.
- ☑ Try not to contaminate with saliva or sinus drainage.
- ☑ Collect before starting antibiotics.

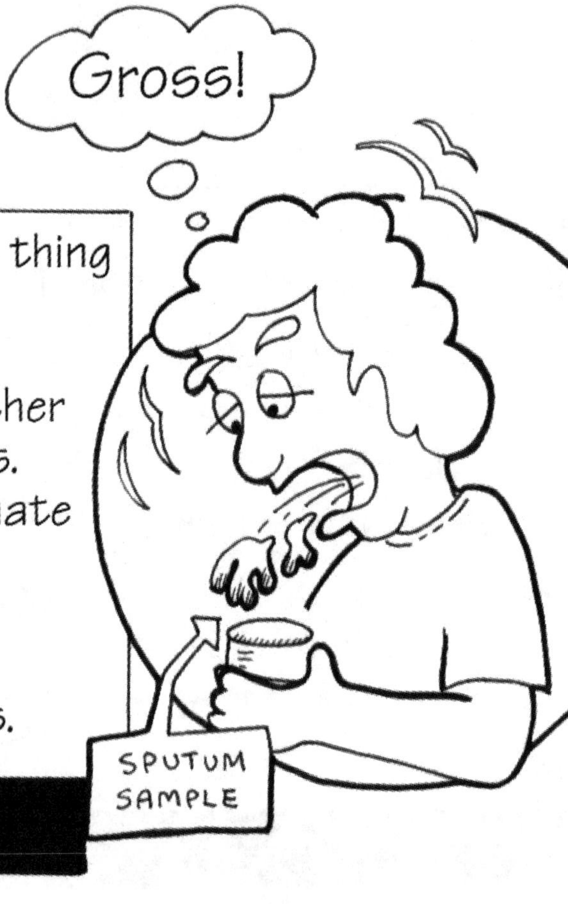

Gross!
SPUTUM SAMPLE
CJMILLER

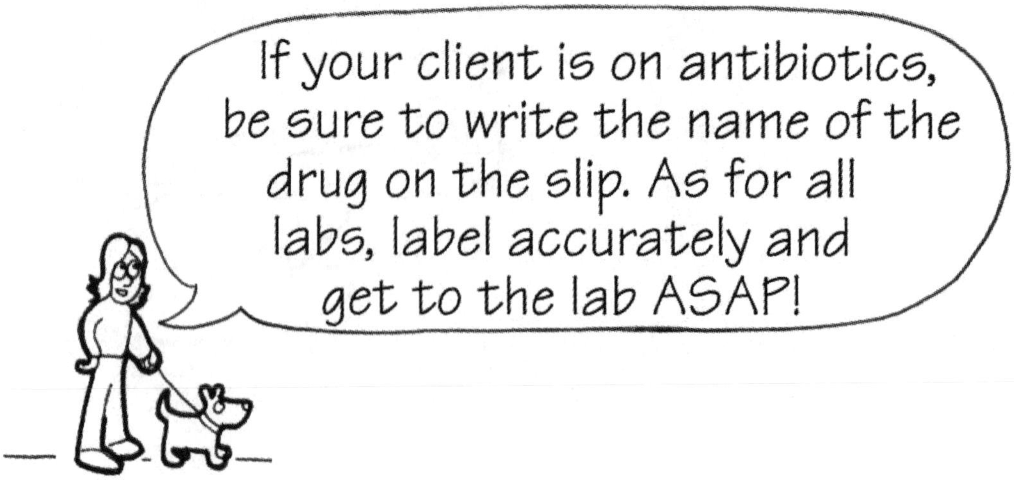

If your client is on antibiotics, be sure to write the name of the drug on the slip. As for all labs, label accurately and get to the lab ASAP!

STOOL 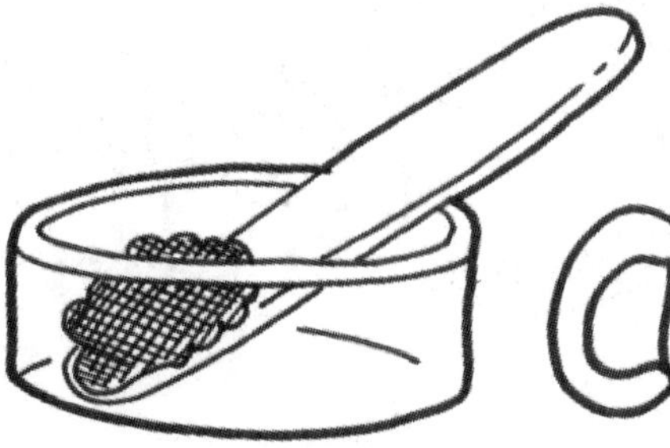 CULTURES

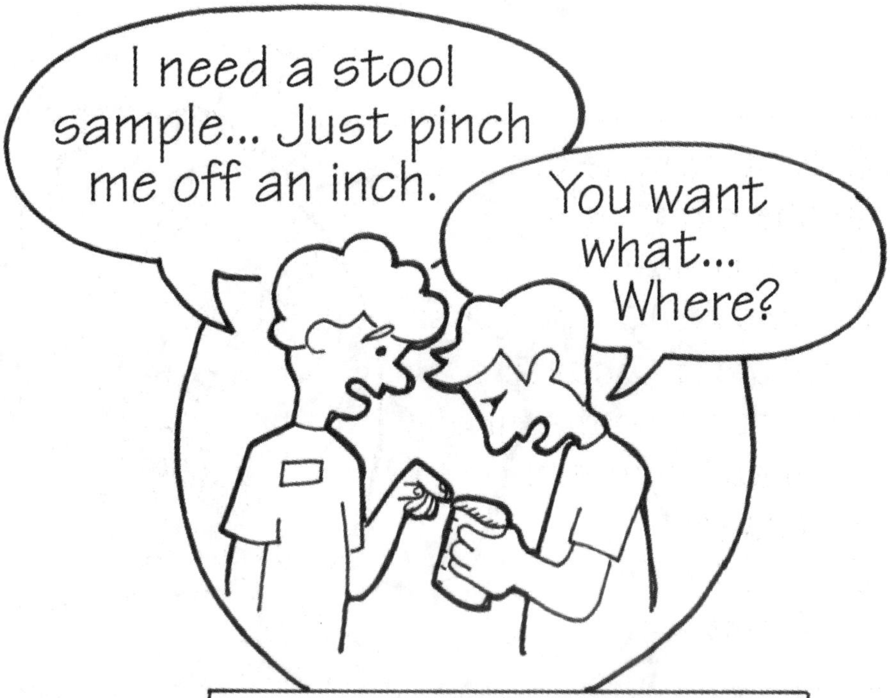
I need a stool sample... Just pinch me off an inch.
You want what... Where?

- ☑ Use a "collection hat" to catch the specimen.
- ☑ You need about an inch of stool which you or the client can collect using a sterile tongue blade.
- ☑ Place specimen in a sterile container; try to keep it free from urine.

C.MILLER

THROAT CULTURES

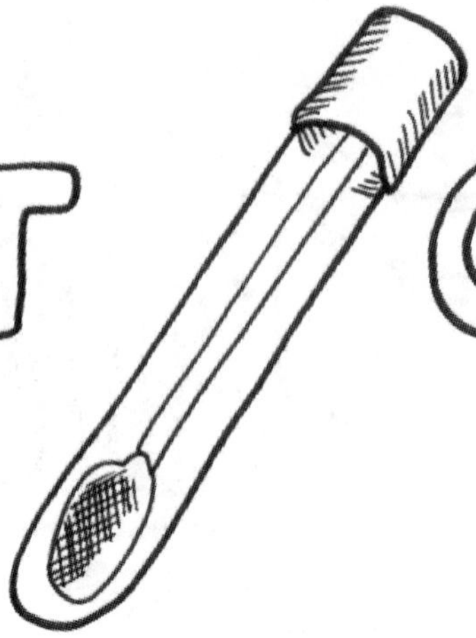

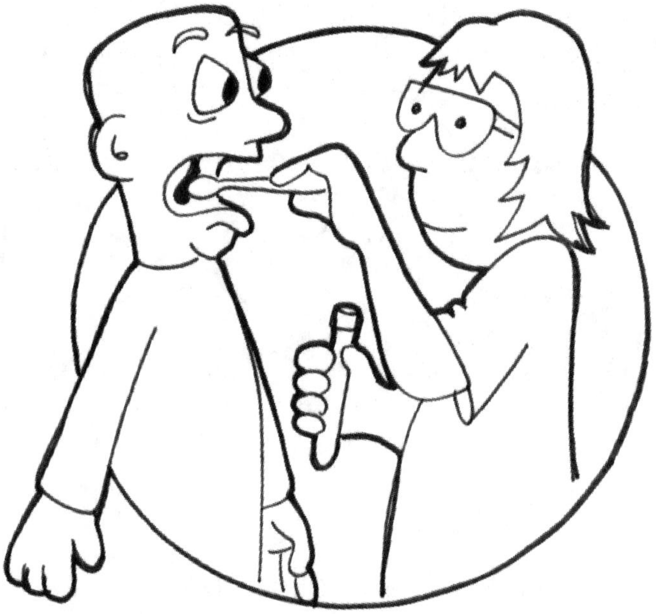

- ☑ Collect culture prior to starting antibiotics.
- ☑ Swab the inflammed or ulcerated area of the throat.
- ☑ Place swab or applicator in culturette tube with it's medium.
- ☑ If client is on an antibiotic, write the name of the drug on the lab slip.
- ☑ Label specimen appropriately.

C. MILLER

URINE CULTURES

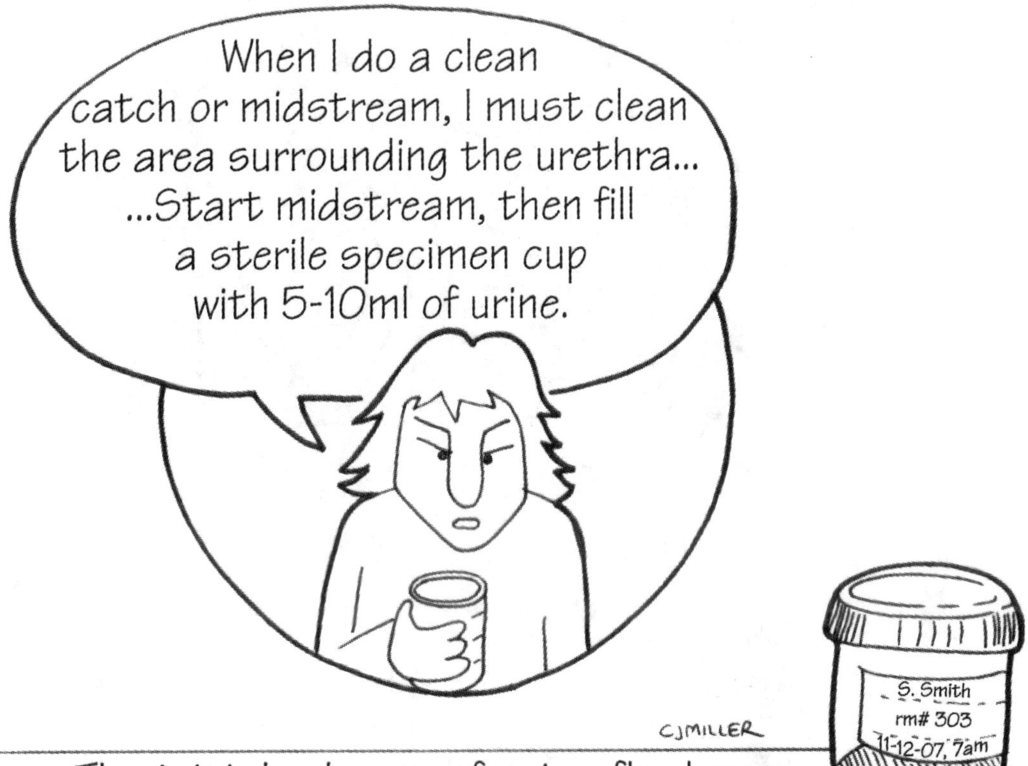
When I do a clean catch or midstream, I must clean the area surrounding the urethra... ...Start midstream, then fill a sterile specimen cup with 5-10ml of urine.
S. Smith
rm# 303
11-12-07, 7am
CJMILLER

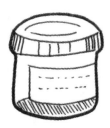

The initial release of urine flushes the urethra. The test is best done on the first morning voiding and the specimen needs to go to the lab immediately.

Label Accurately!!!!

WOUND CULTURES

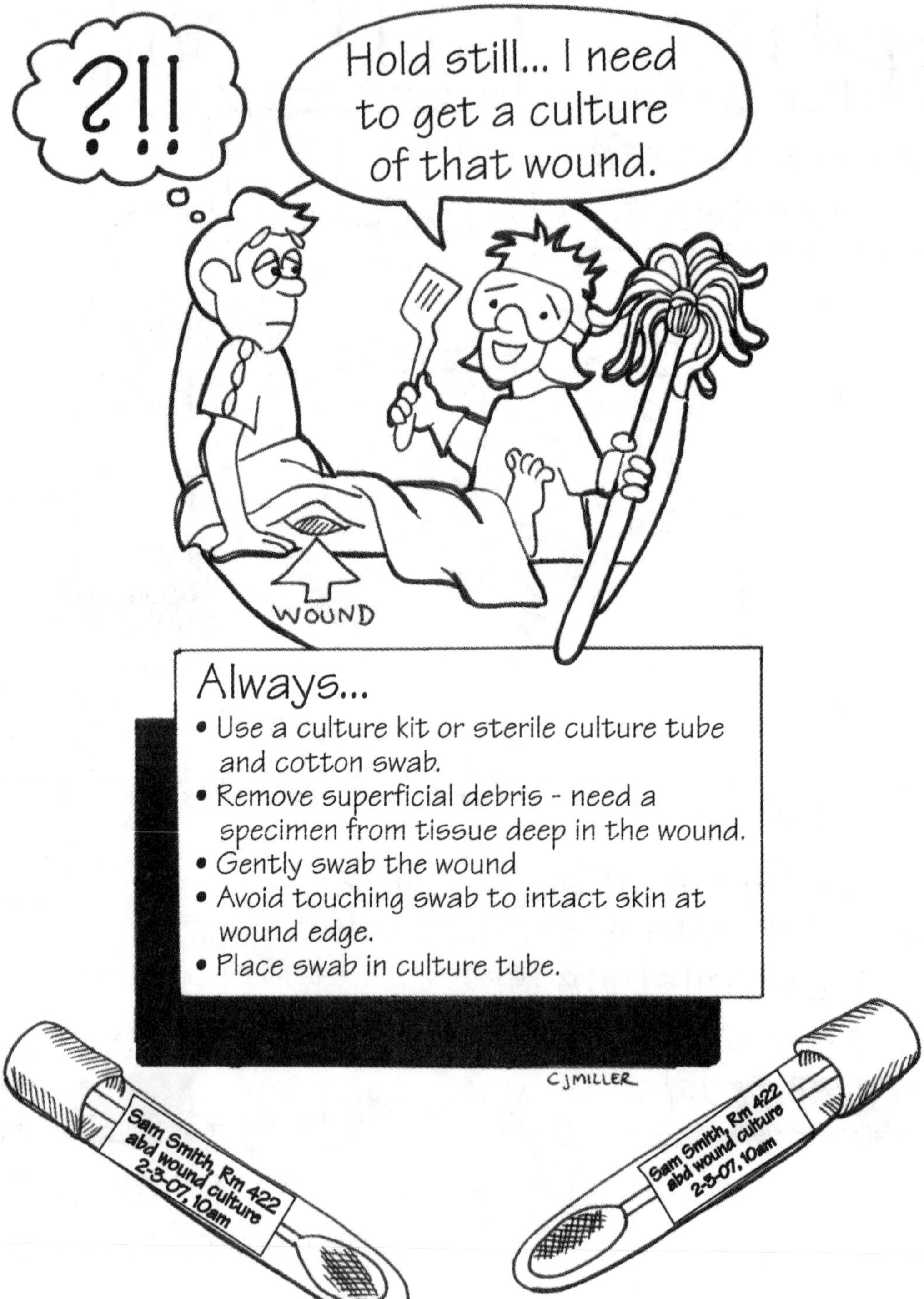
?!!
Hold still... I need to get a culture of that wound.
WOUND
Always...
• Use a culture kit or sterile culture tube and cotton swab.
• Remove superficial debris - need a specimen from tissue deep in the wound.
• Gently swab the wound
• Avoid touching swab to intact skin at wound edge.
• Place swab in culture tube.
CJMILLER
Sam Smith, Rm 422 abd wound culture 2-3-07, 10am
Sam Smith, Rm 422 abd wound culture 2-3-07, 10am

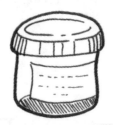

Ammonia Level

(Adult 10-80 mcg/dl)

Ammonia is a byproduct of protein break down by the liver, which then converts ammonia to urea and excretes it.

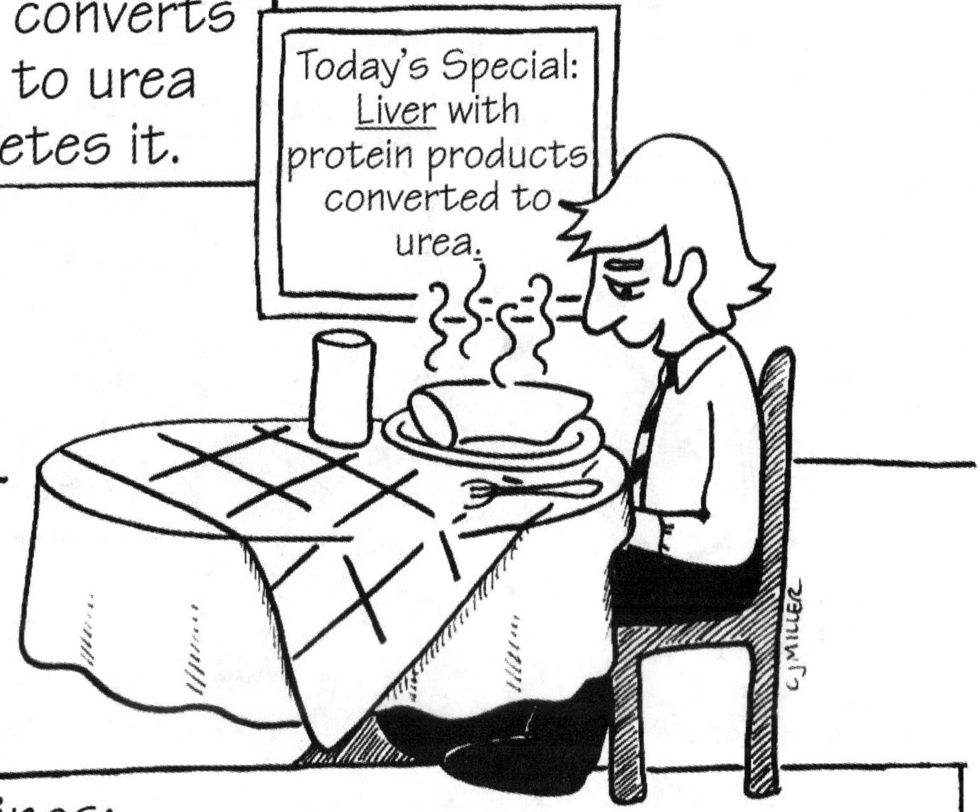
Today's Special:
Liver with protein products converted to urea.
CJMILLER

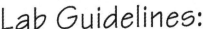

Lab Guidelines:

- No smoking for several hours prior to test.
- Draw 5-7ml in a green top tube.
- Get blood to lab on ice.
- High levels of ammonia occur with liver problems.

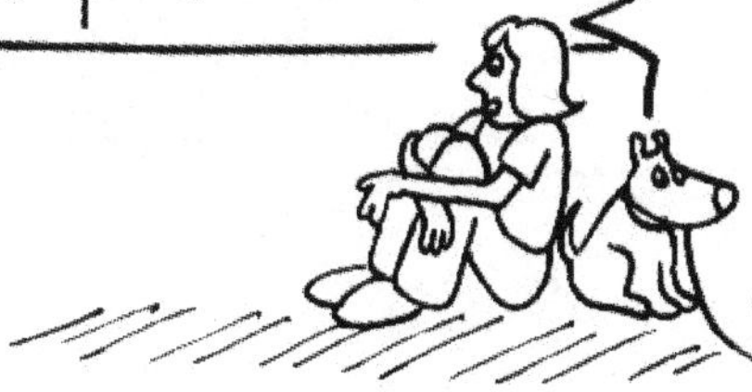

Drugs that could alter the test are antibiotics, alcohol, potassium salts.

Blood Urea Nitrogen (BUN)

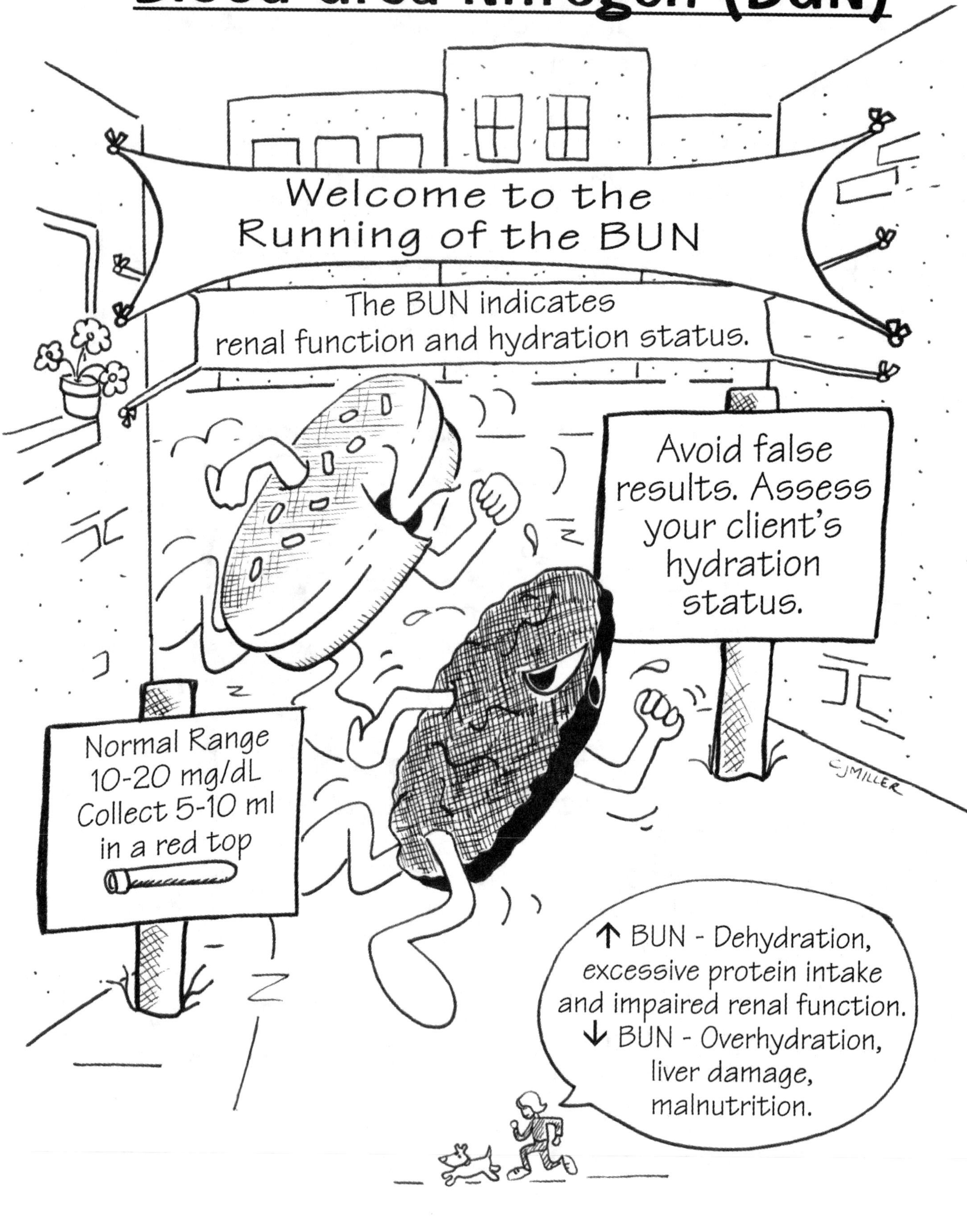

Welcome to the Running of the BUN
The BUN indicates renal function and hydration status.
Avoid false results. Assess your client's hydration status.
Normal Range 10-20 mg/dL Collect 5-10 ml in a red top
↑ BUN - Dehydration, excessive protein intake and impaired renal function.
↓ BUN - Overhydration, liver damage, malnutrition.
CJMILLER

Creatinine & Creatinine Clearance

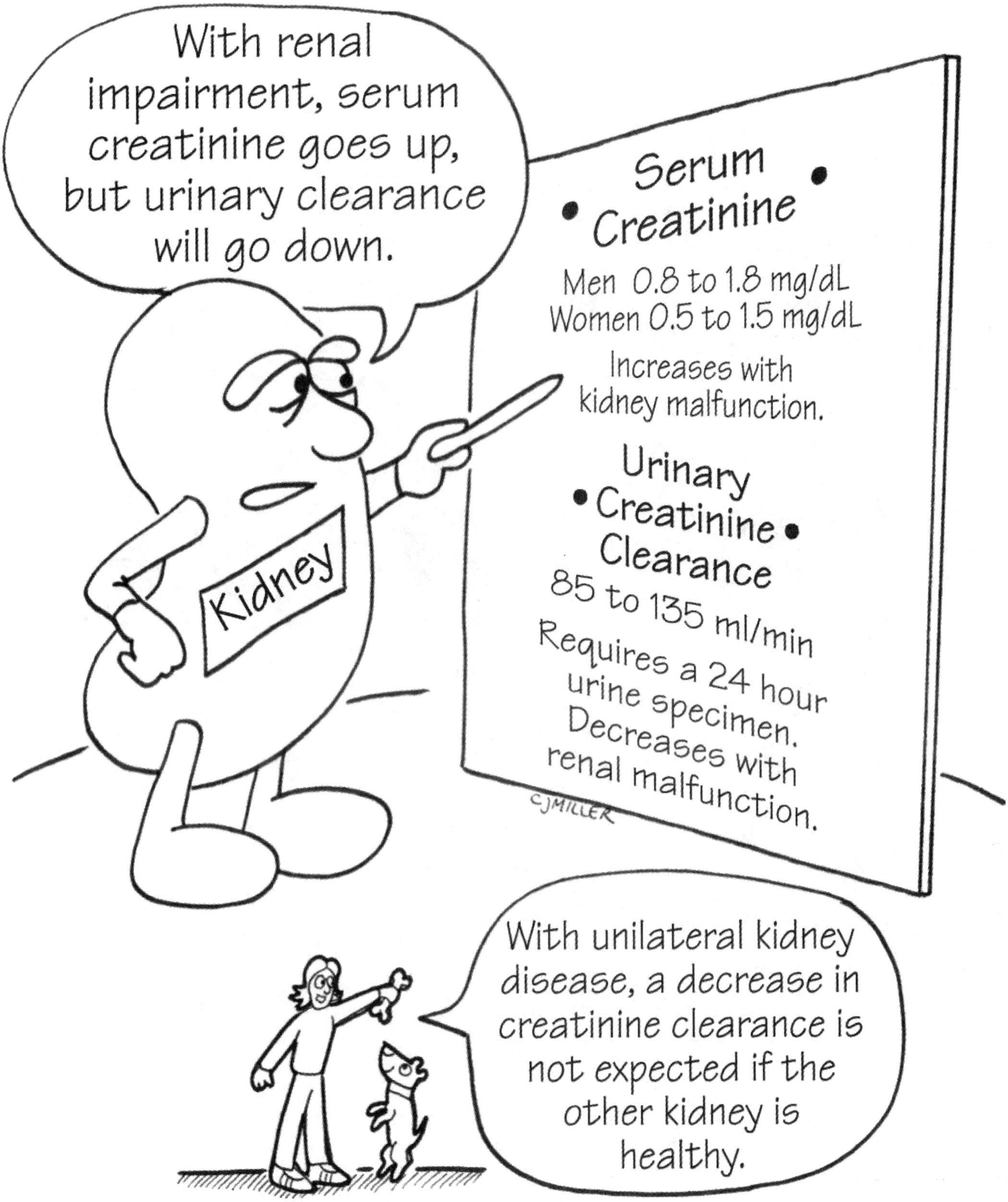

With renal impairment, serum creatinine goes up, but urinary clearance will go down.
Serum Creatinine
Men 0.8 to 1.8 mg/dL
Women 0.5 to 1.5 mg/dL
Increases with kidney malfunction.
Urinary Creatinine Clearance
85 to 135 ml/min
Requires a 24 hour urine specimen.
Decreases with renal malfunction.
Kidney
CJMILLER
With unilateral kidney disease, a decrease in creatinine clearance is not expected if the other kidney is healthy.

Fibrinogen

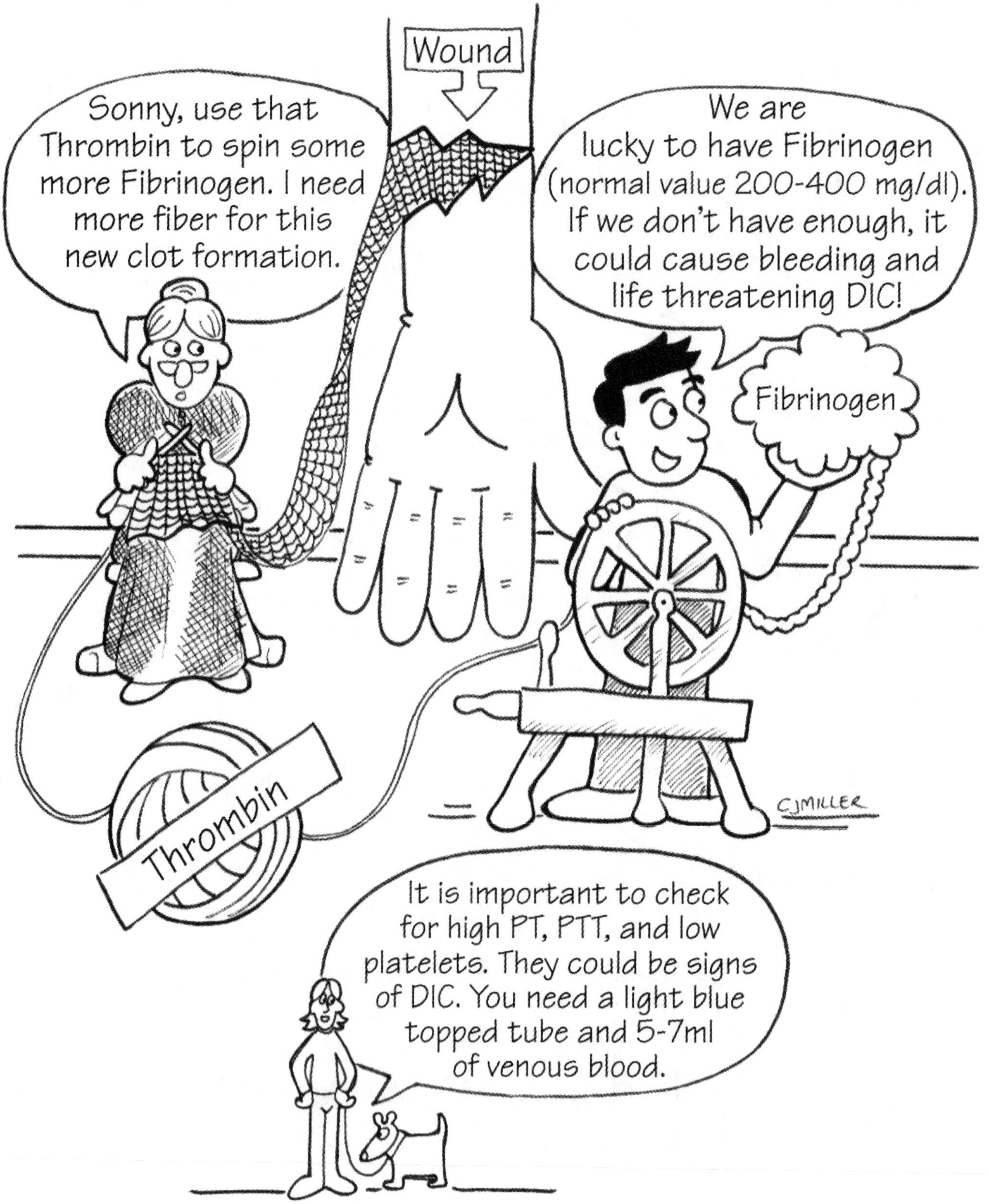
Wound
Sonny, use that Thrombin to spin some more Fibrinogen. I need more fiber for this new clot formation.
We are lucky to have Fibrinogen (normal value 200-400 mg/dl). If we don't have enough, it could cause bleeding and life threatening DIC!
Fibrinogen
Thrombin
CJMILLER
It is important to check for high PT, PTT, and low platelets. They could be signs of DIC. You need a light blue topped tube and 5-7ml of venous blood.

Gamma-Glutamyl Transferase (GGT)

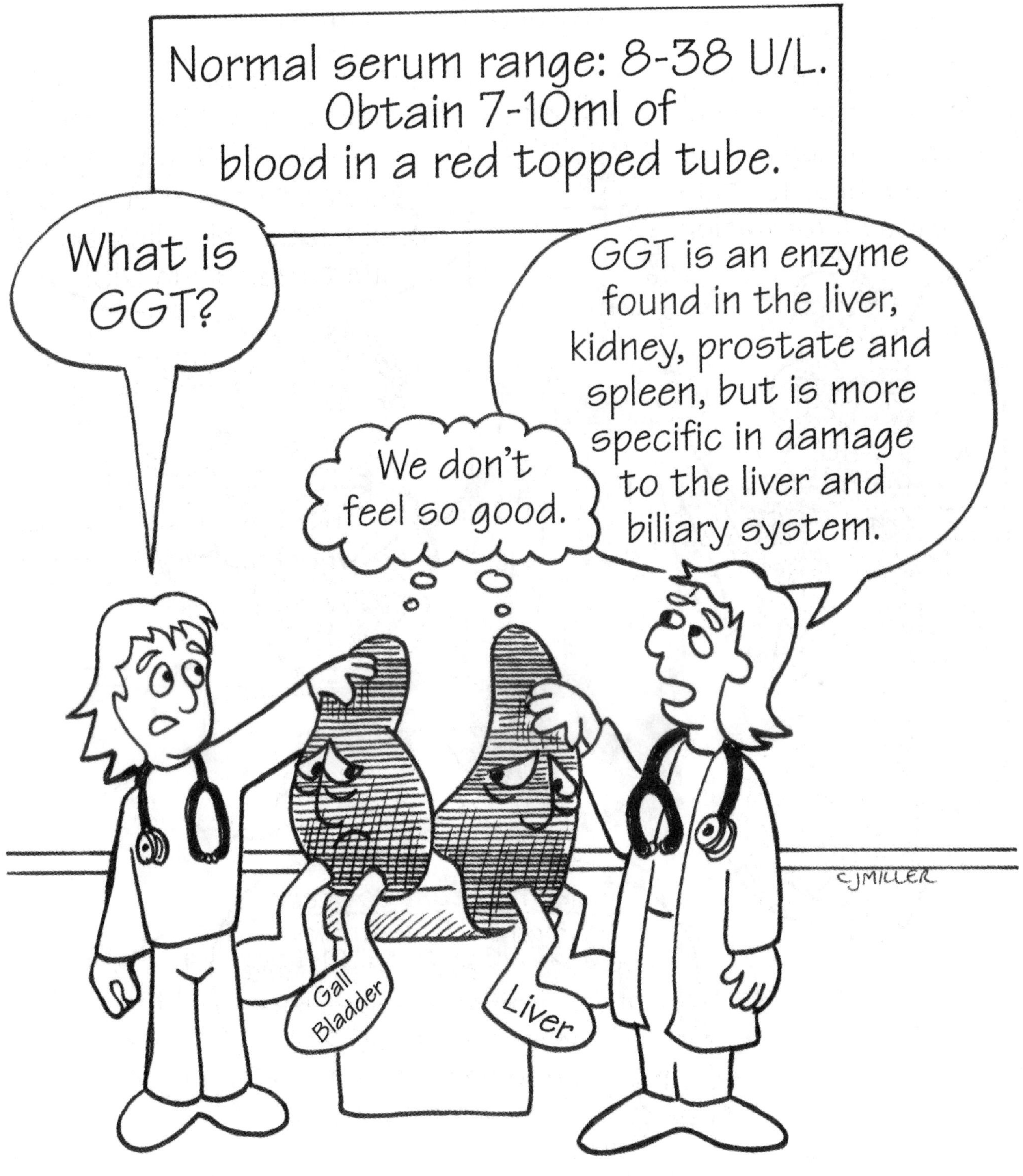
Normal serum range: 8-38 U/L. Obtain 7-10ml of blood in a red topped tube.
What is GGT?
We don't feel so good.
GGT is an enzyme found in the liver, kidney, prostate and spleen, but is more specific in damage to the liver and biliary system.
Gall Bladder
Liver
CJMILLER

Hematocrit

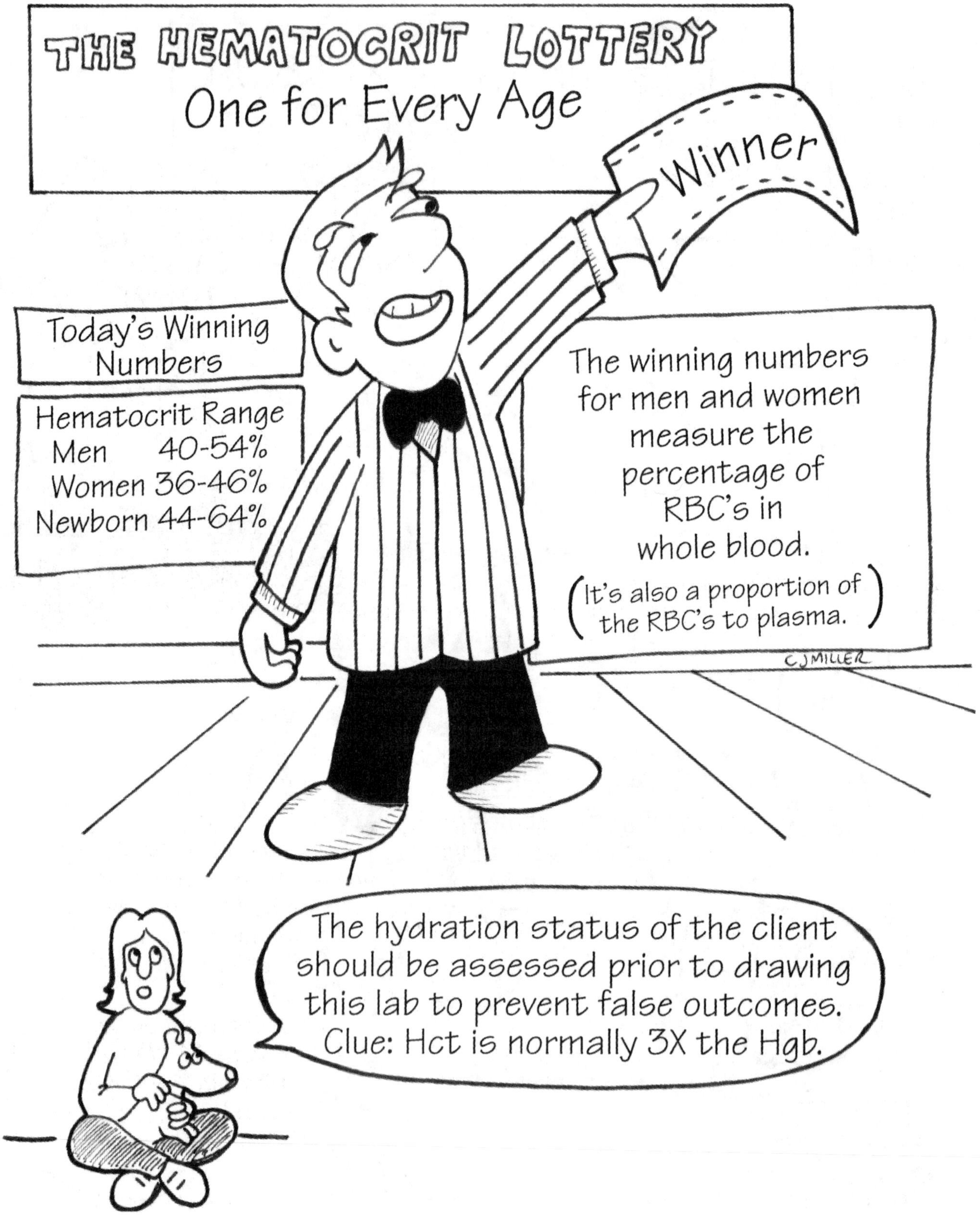
THE HEMATOCRIT LOTTERY
One for Every Age
Winner
Today's Winning Numbers
Hematocrit Range
Men 40-54%
Women 36-46%
Newborn 44-64%
The winning numbers for men and women measure the percentage of RBC's in whole blood.
(It's also a proportion of the RBC's to plasma.)
CJMILLER
The hydration status of the client should be assessed prior to drawing this lab to prevent false outcomes. Clue: Hct is normally 3X the Hgb.

Hemoglobin

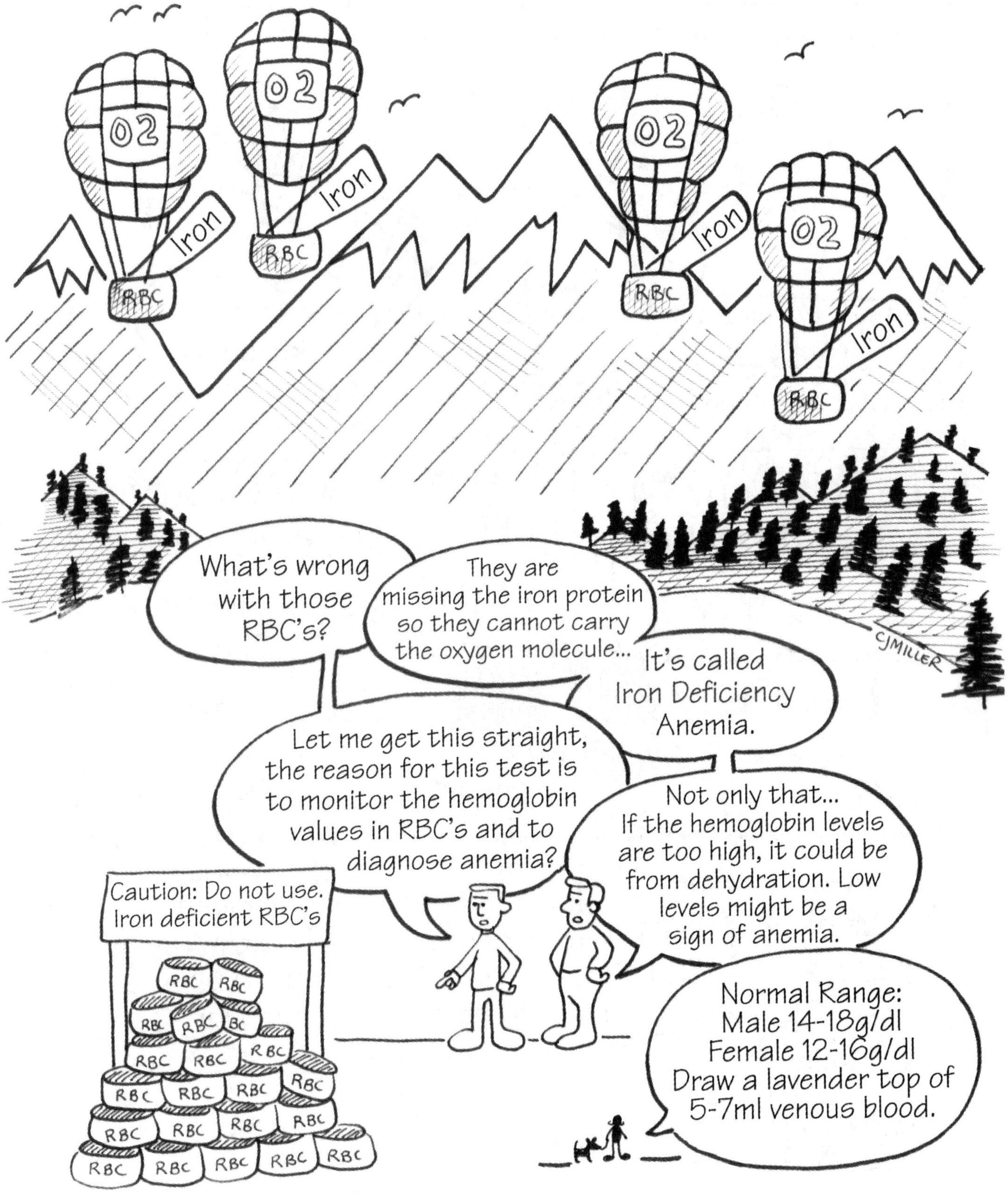
O2
Iron
RBC
What's wrong with those RBC's?
They are missing the iron protein so they cannot carry the oxygen molecule...
It's called Iron Deficiency Anemia.
Let me get this straight, the reason for this test is to monitor the hemoglobin values in RBC's and to diagnose anemia?
Not only that... If the hemoglobin levels are too high, it could be from dehydration. Low levels might be a sign of anemia.
Caution: Do not use. Iron deficient RBC's
Normal Range: Male 14-18g/dl Female 12-16g/dl Draw a lavender top of 5-7ml venous blood.
CJMILLER

Lipoproteins

If It Tastes Good, It's Probably Bad For You!

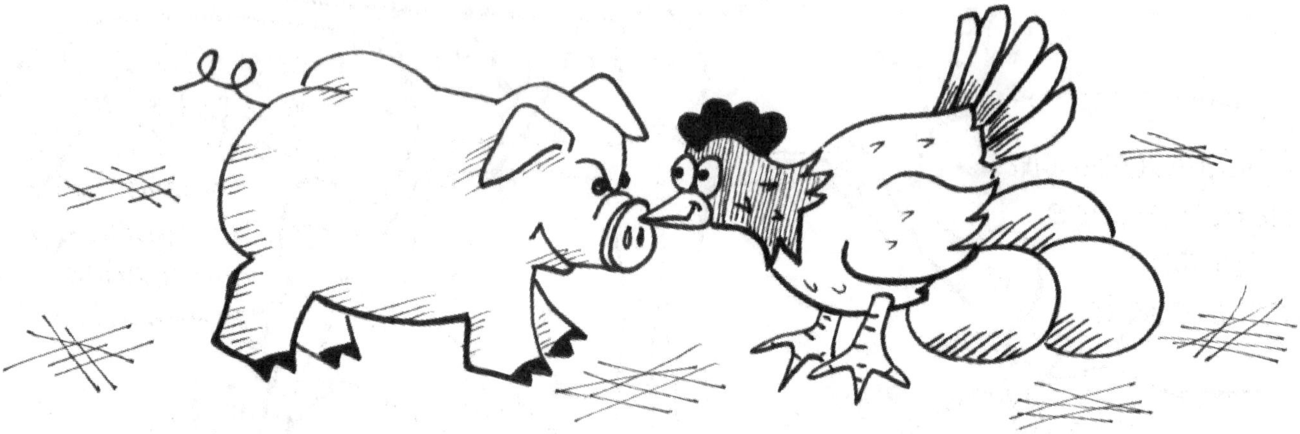

Low Density Lipoproteins...	High Density Lipoproteins...
(>130mg/dl) increases risk of development of coronary artery disease.	(>60mg/dl) are Good For You

CJMILLER

Warning: This is a 12 to 14 hour fast (except water) and no alcoholic beverages for 24 hours before test. Draw 5-7ml in Red Top

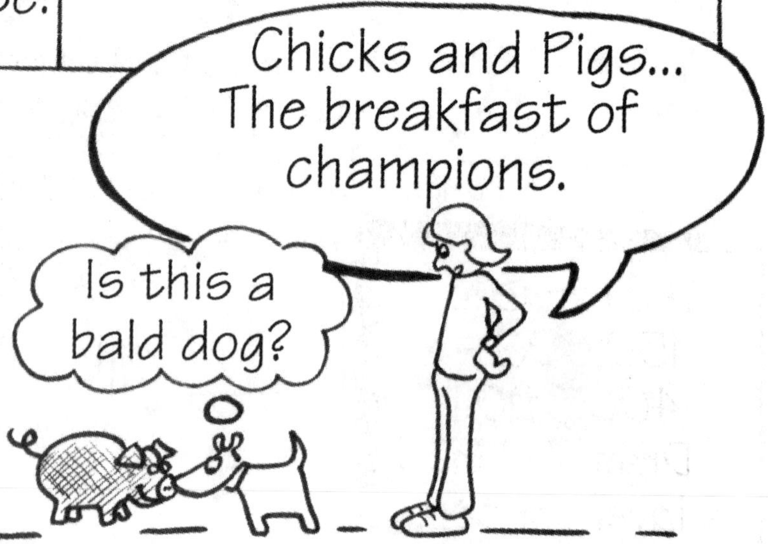
Chicks and Pigs... The breakfast of champions.
Is this a bald dog?

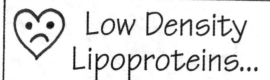

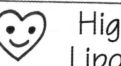

Platelet Count

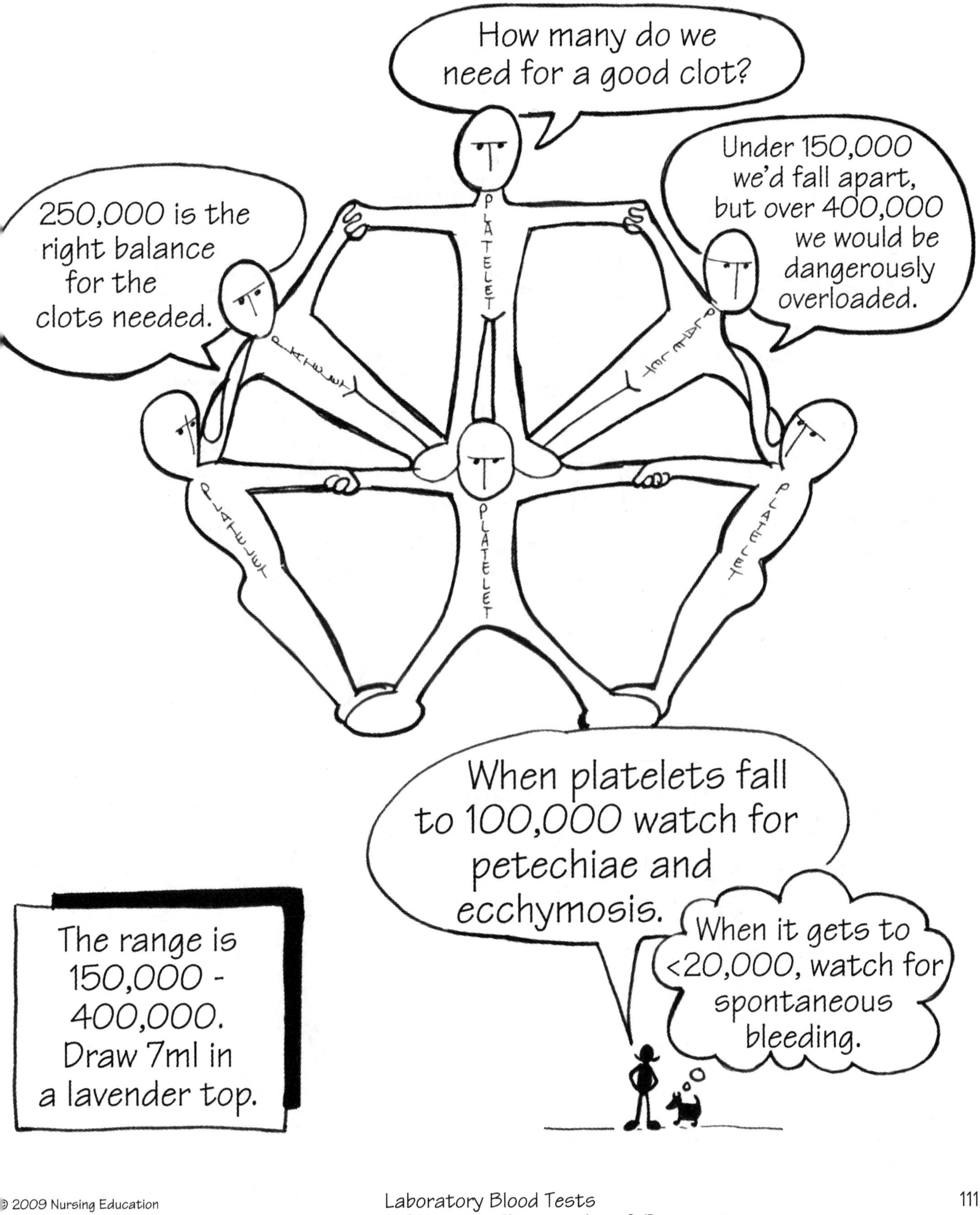

How many do we need for a good clot?
250,000 is the right balance for the clots needed.
Under 150,000 we'd fall apart, but over 400,000 we would be dangerously overloaded.
PLATELET
PLATELET
When platelets fall to 100,000 watch for petechiae and ecchymosis.
When it gets to <20,000, watch for spontaneous bleeding.
The range is 150,000 - 400,000. Draw 7ml in a lavender top.

Potassium (Serum)

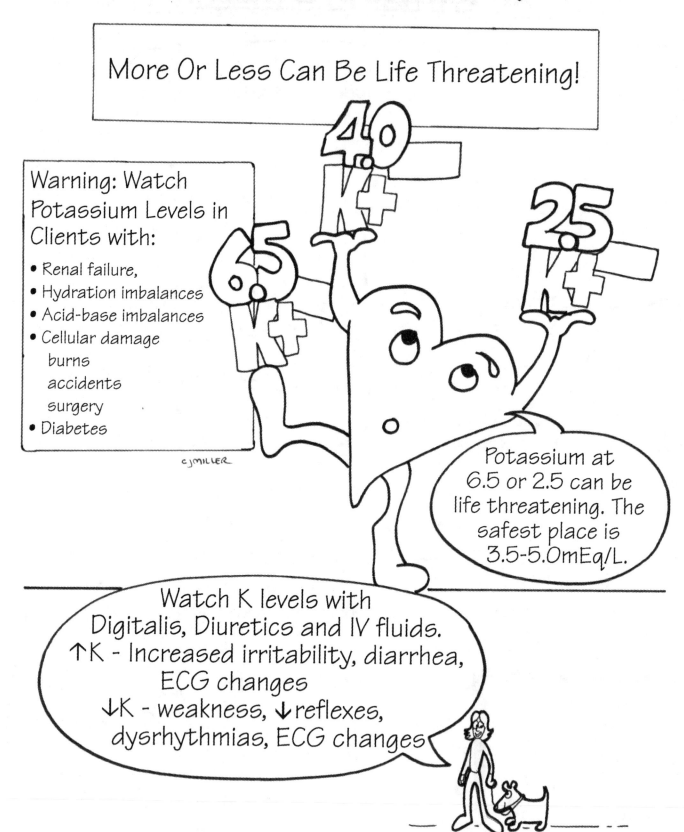

More Or Less Can Be Life Threatening!

Warning: Watch Potassium Levels in Clients with:

- Renal failure,
- Hydration imbalances
- Acid-base imbalances
- Cellular damage
  - burns
  - accidents
  - surgery
- Diabetes

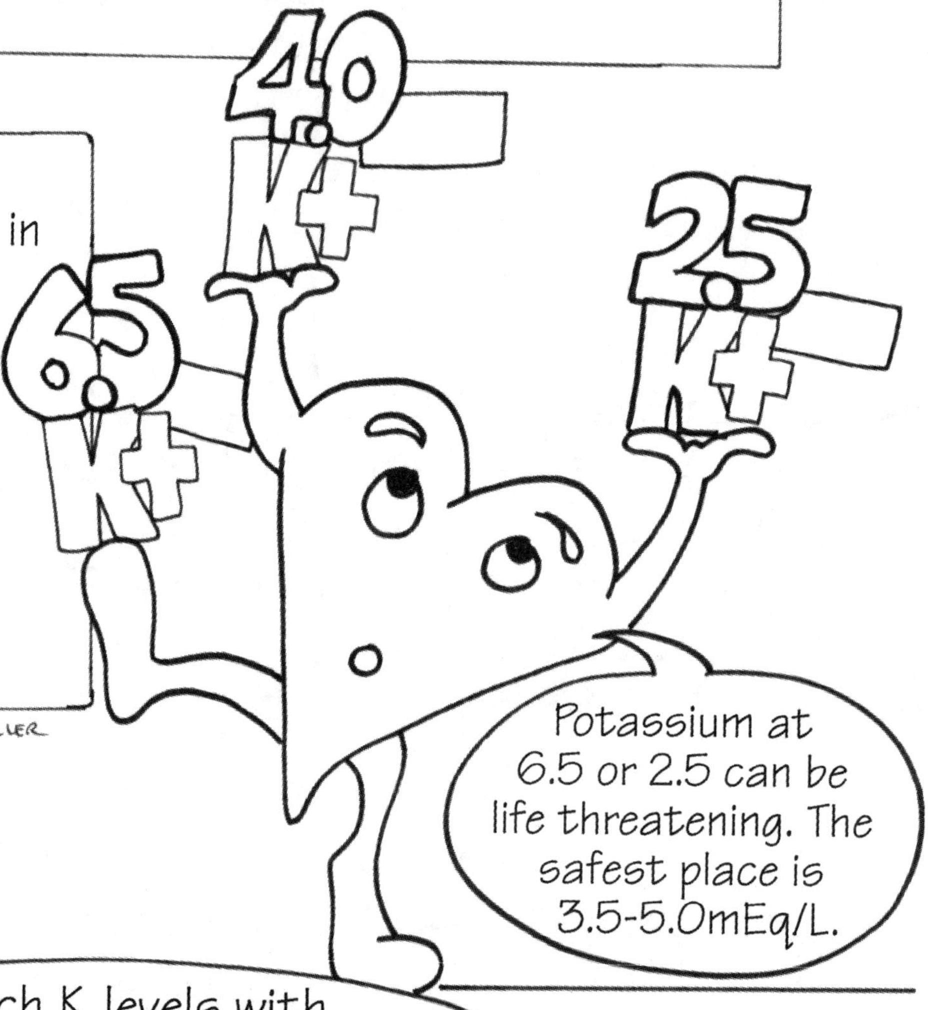
4.0 K+
6.5 K+
2.5 K+
CJMILLER
Potassium at 6.5 or 2.5 can be life threatening. The safest place is 3.5-5.0mEq/L.

Watch K levels with
Digitalis, Diuretics and IV fluids.
↑K - Increased irritability, diarrhea, ECG changes
↓K - weakness, ↓reflexes, dysrhythmias, ECG changes

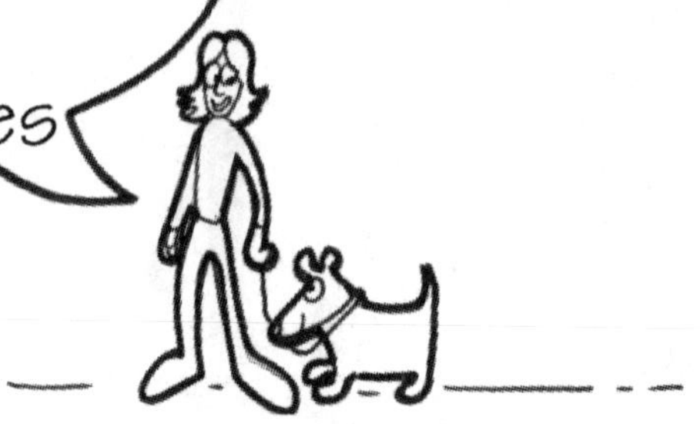

Prostatic Specific Antigen (PSA)

It's a guy thing for those with a prostate.

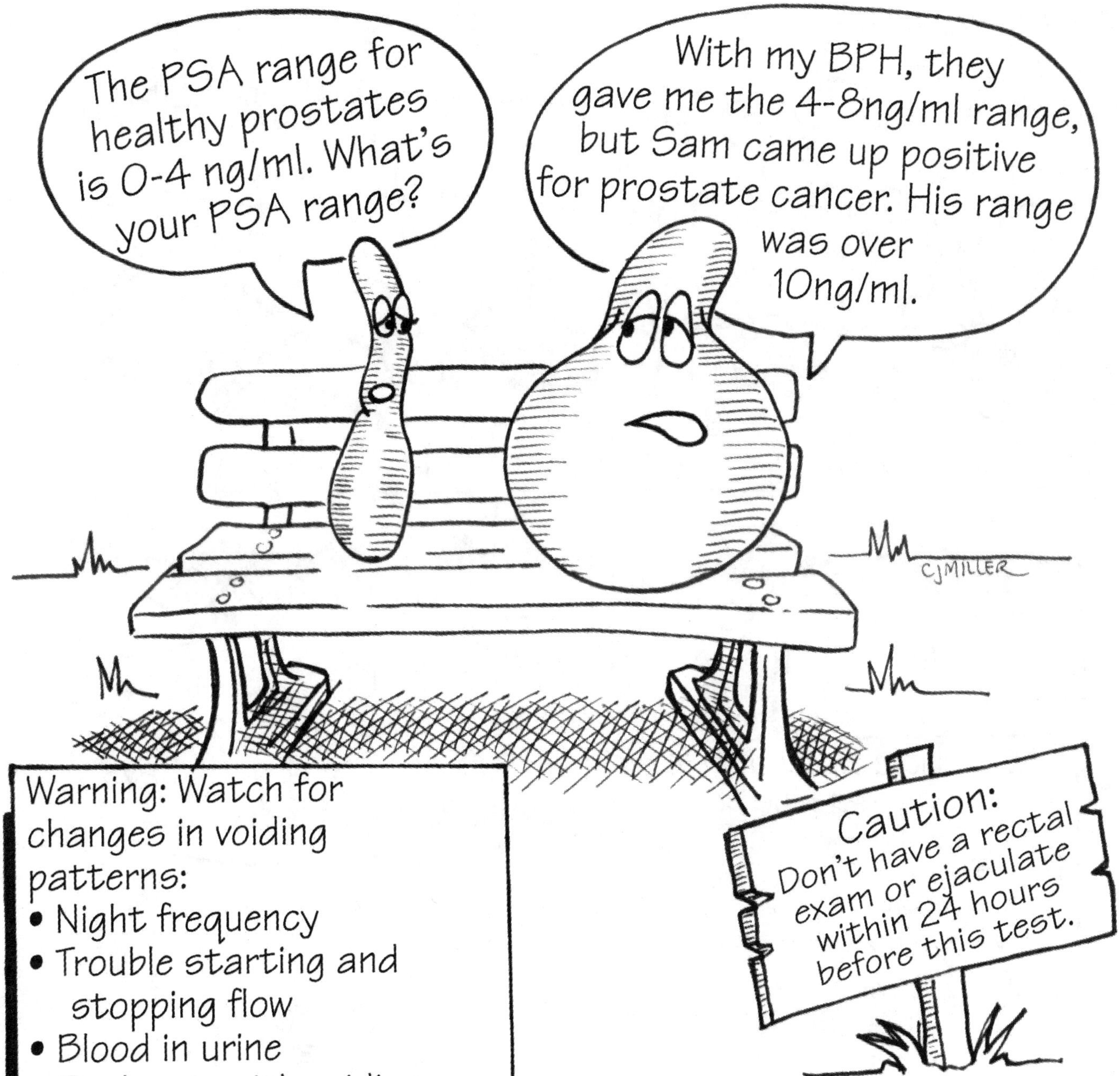
The PSA range for healthy prostates is 0-4 ng/ml. What's your PSA range?
With my BPH, they gave me the 4-8ng/ml range, but Sam came up positive for prostate cancer. His range was over 10ng/ml.
CJMILLER
Caution: Don't have a rectal exam or ejaculate within 24 hours before this test.

Warning: Watch for changes in voiding patterns:
- Night frequency
- Trouble starting and stopping flow
- Blood in urine
- Back pain with voiding

Prothrombin Time (PT) and INR

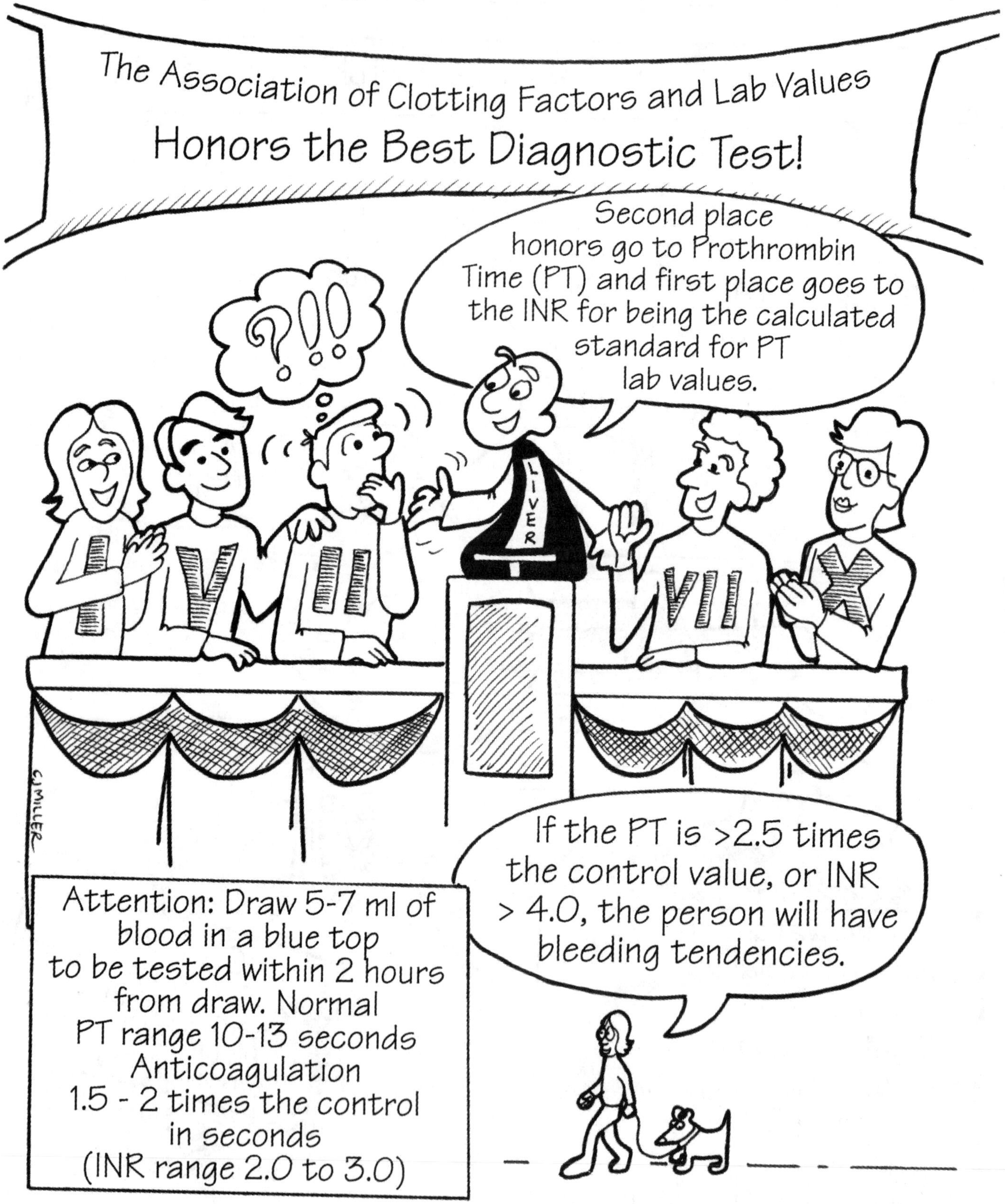

The Association of Clotting Factors and Lab Values
Honors the Best Diagnostic Test!
?!!
Second place honors go to Prothrombin Time (PT) and first place goes to the INR for being the calculated standard for PT lab values.
LIVER
I
V
II
VII
X
C.J.MILLER
If the PT is >2.5 times the control value, or INR > 4.0, the person will have bleeding tendencies.
Attention: Draw 5-7 ml of blood in a blue top to be tested within 2 hours from draw. Normal PT range 10-13 seconds Anticoagulation 1.5 - 2 times the control in seconds (INR range 2.0 to 3.0)

PTT and APTT

"A Time and Place To Bleed"

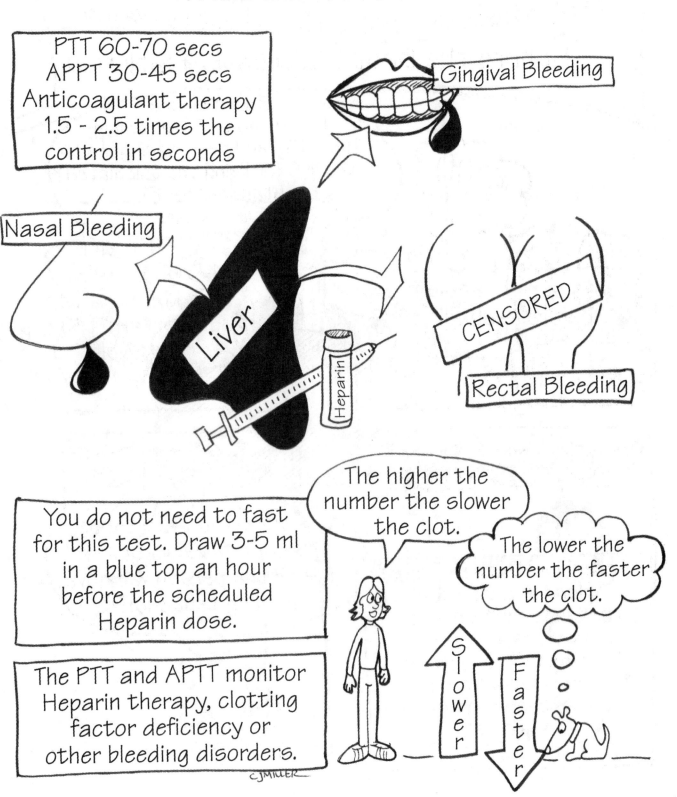

PTT 60-70 secs
APPT 30-45 secs
Anticoagulant therapy 1.5 - 2.5 times the control in seconds

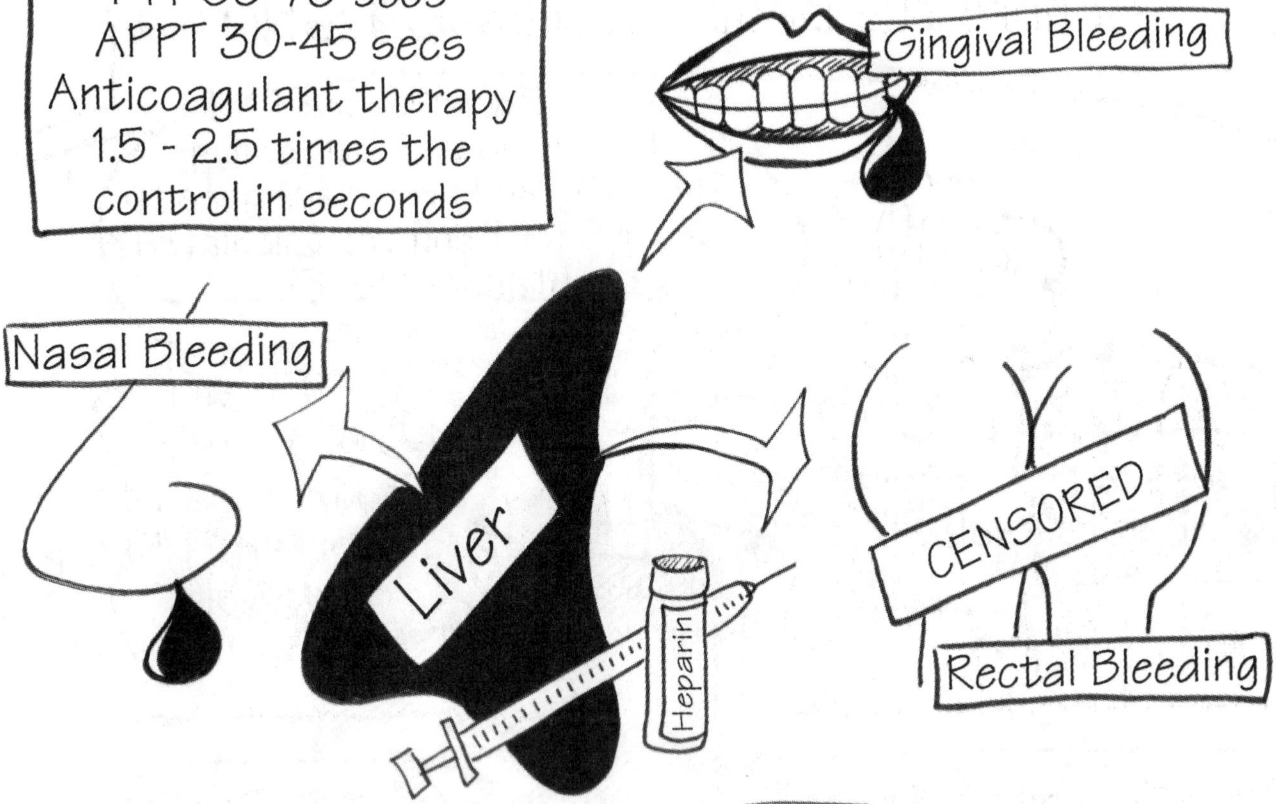

Gingival Bleeding
Nasal Bleeding
Liver
Heparin
CENSORED
Rectal Bleeding

You do not need to fast for this test. Draw 3-5 ml in a blue top an hour before the scheduled Heparin dose.

The PTT and APTT monitor Heparin therapy, clotting factor deficiency or other bleeding disorders.

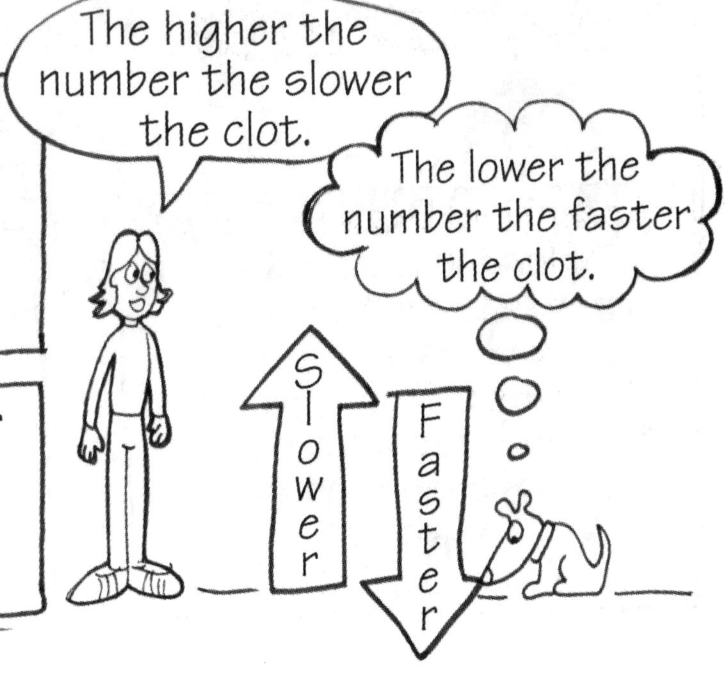

The higher the number the slower the clot.
The lower the number the faster the clot.
Slower
Faster
CJMILLER

Digoxin Level

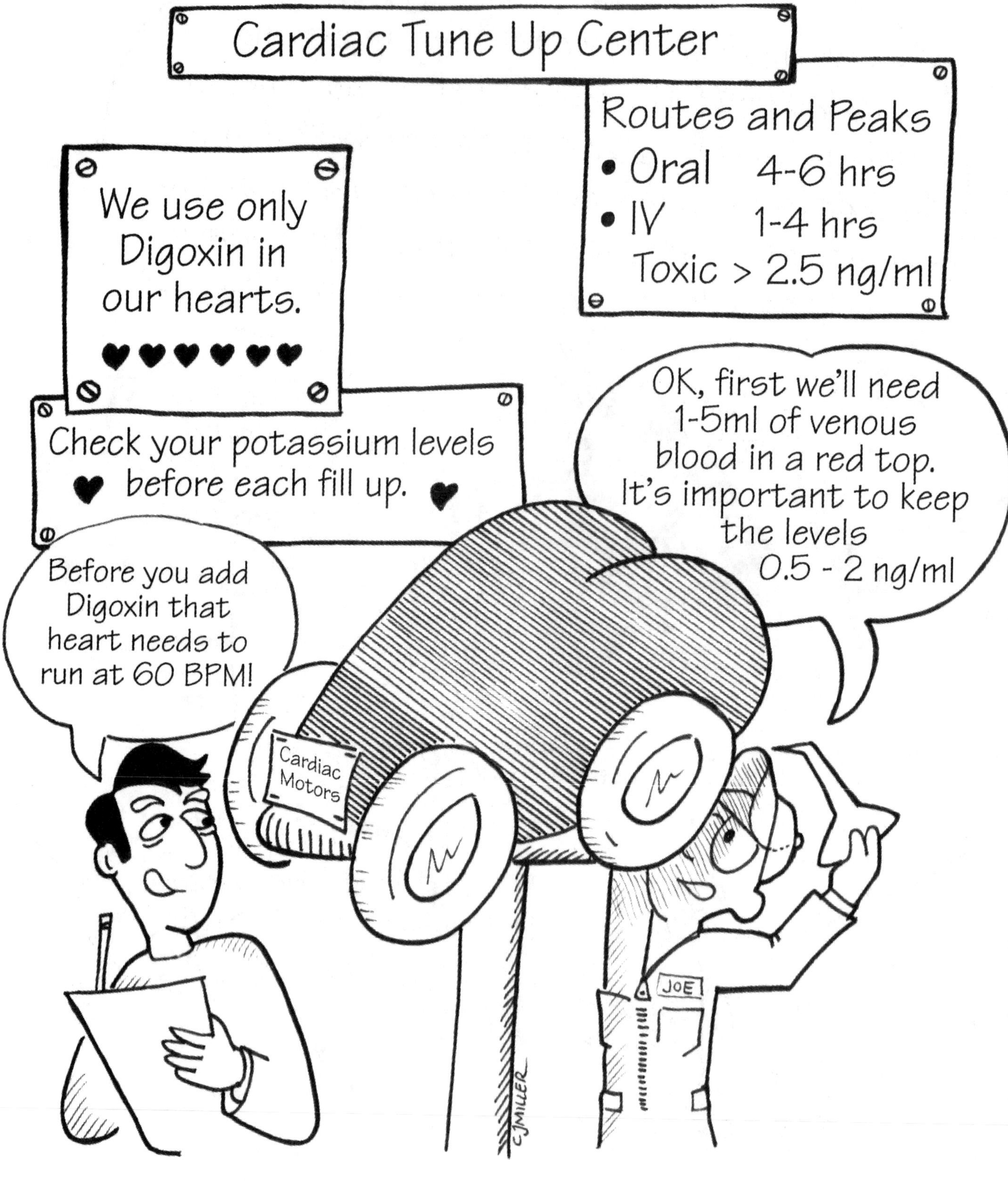
Cardiac Tune Up Center
Routes and Peaks
• Oral 4-6 hrs
• IV 1-4 hrs
Toxic > 2.5 ng/ml
We use only Digoxin in our hearts.
Check your potassium levels before each fill up.
OK, first we'll need 1-5ml of venous blood in a red top. It's important to keep the levels 0.5 - 2 ng/ml
Before you add Digoxin that heart needs to run at 60 BPM!
Cardiac Motors
JOE
CJMILLER

Lipase and Amylase (Serum)

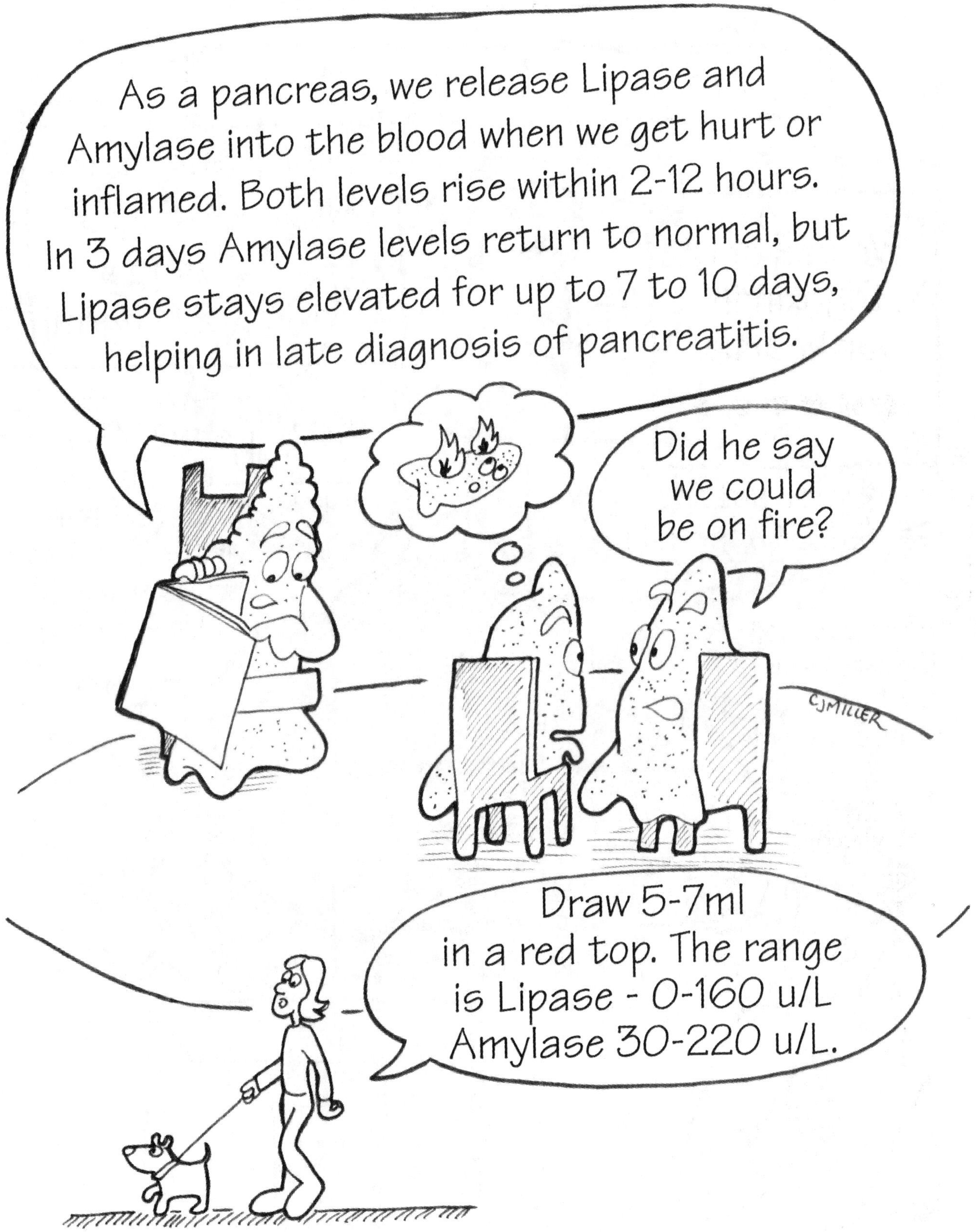

As a pancreas, we release Lipase and Amylase into the blood when we get hurt or inflamed. Both levels rise within 2-12 hours. In 3 days Amylase levels return to normal, but Lipase stays elevated for up to 7 to 10 days, helping in late diagnosis of pancreatitis.
Did he say we could be on fire?
CJMILLER
Draw 5-7ml in a red top. The range is Lipase - 0-160 u/L Amylase 30-220 u/L.

Sodium and Chloride (Serum)

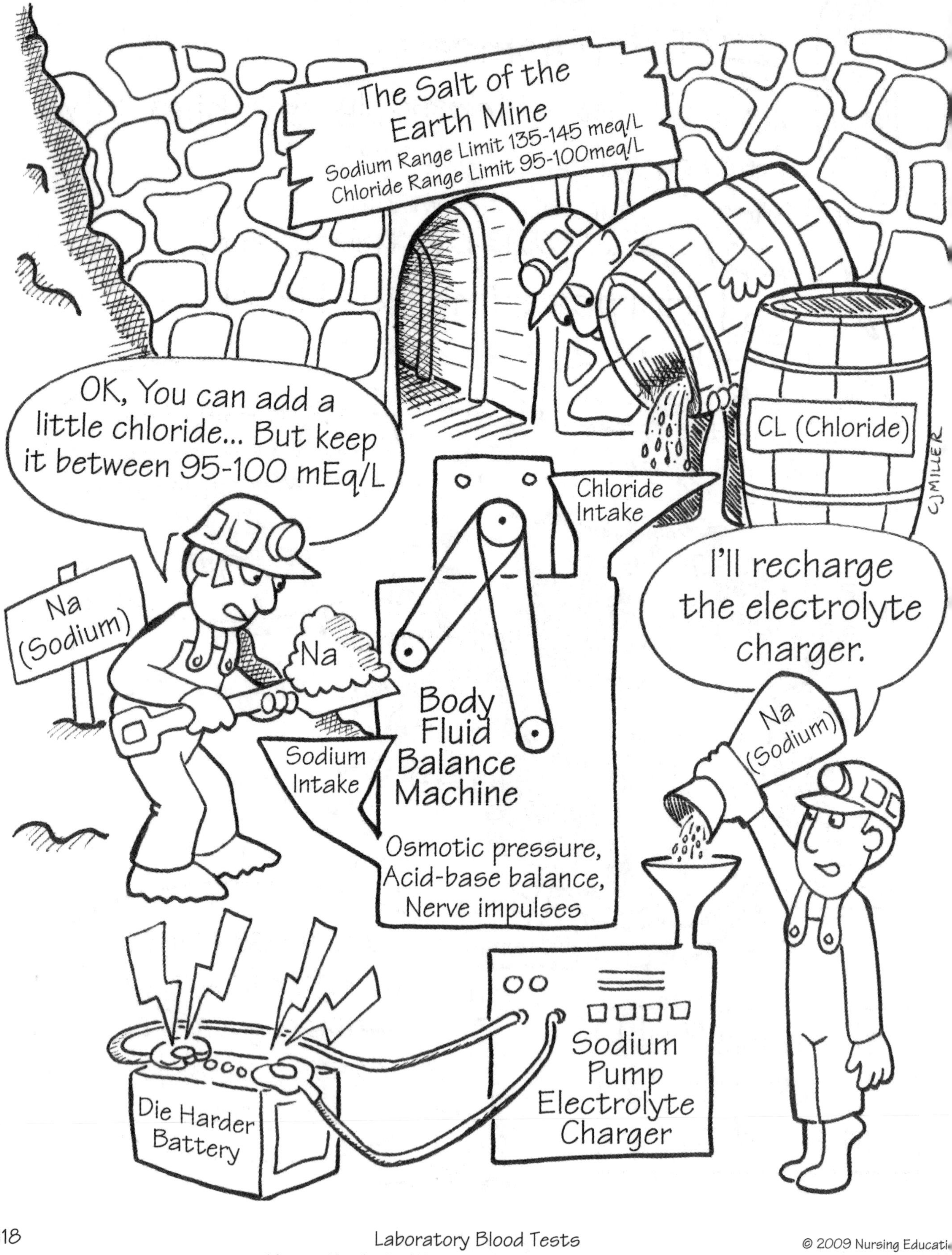

TORCH Screening

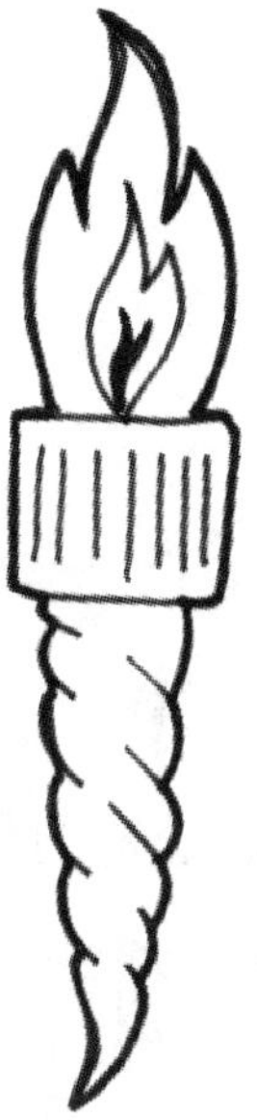

T (Toxoplasmosis)
O (Other - Hepatitis, Syphilis, HIV)
R (Rubella)
C (Cytomegalovirus - CMV)
H (Herpes Simplex - HSV)

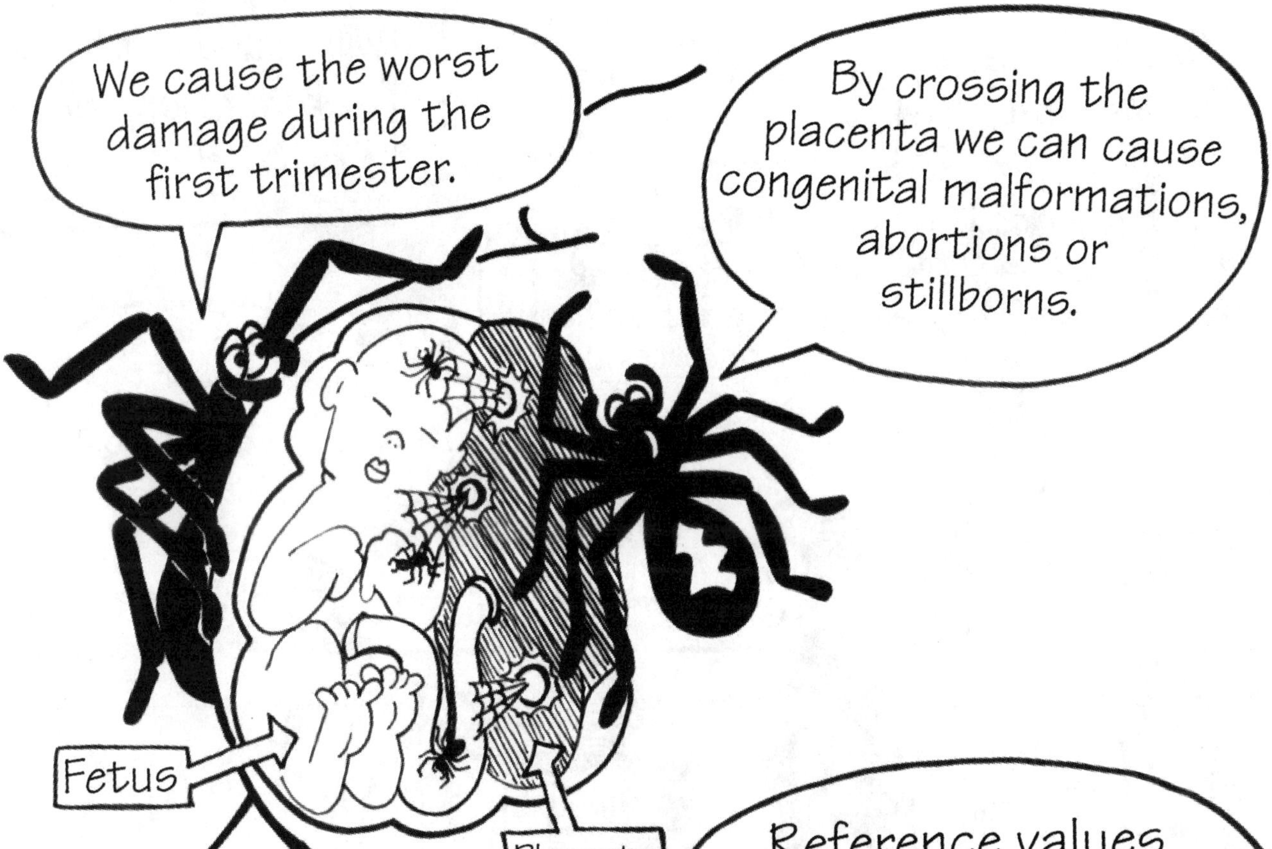

We cause the worst damage during the first trimester.
By crossing the placenta we can cause congenital malformations, abortions or stillborns.
Fetus
Placenta

CJMILLER

You need 7ml of blood in a red top.

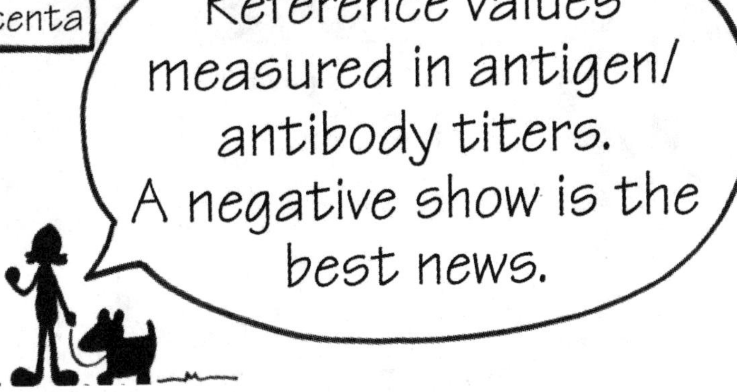

Reference values measured in antigen/ antibody titers. A negative show is the best news.

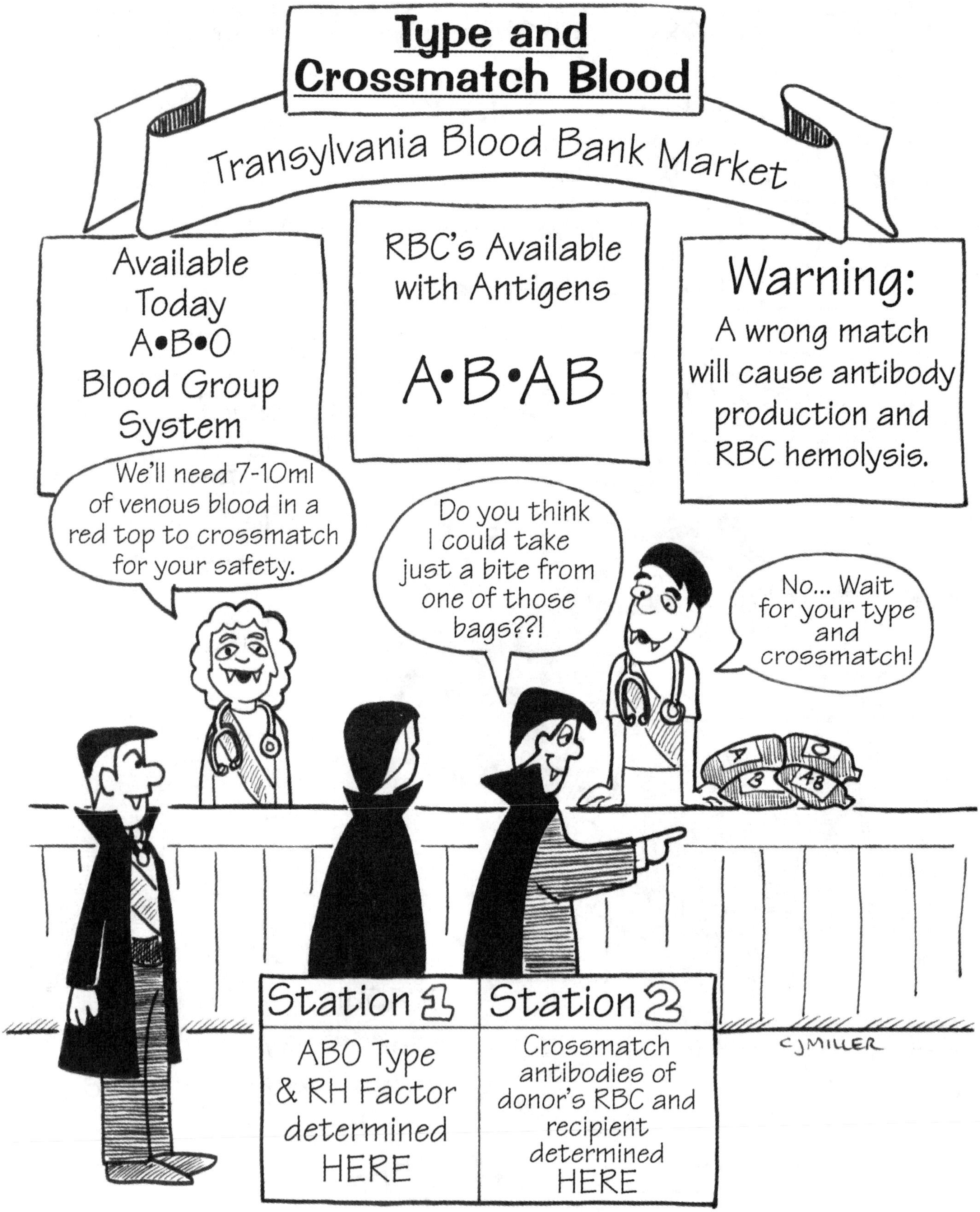
Type and Crossmatch Blood
Transylvania Blood Bank Market
Available Today A•B•O Blood Group System
RBC's Available with Antigens
A•B•AB
Warning:
A wrong match will cause antibody production and RBC hemolysis.
We'll need 7-10ml of venous blood in a red top to crossmatch for your safety.
Do you think I could take just a bite from one of those bags??!
No... Wait for your type and crossmatch!
A
O
B
AB
Station 1
ABO Type & RH Factor determined HERE
Station 2
Crossmatch antibodies of donor's RBC and recipient determined HERE
CJMILLER

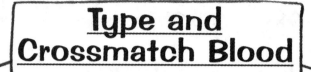

White Blood Cells (WBC) Count

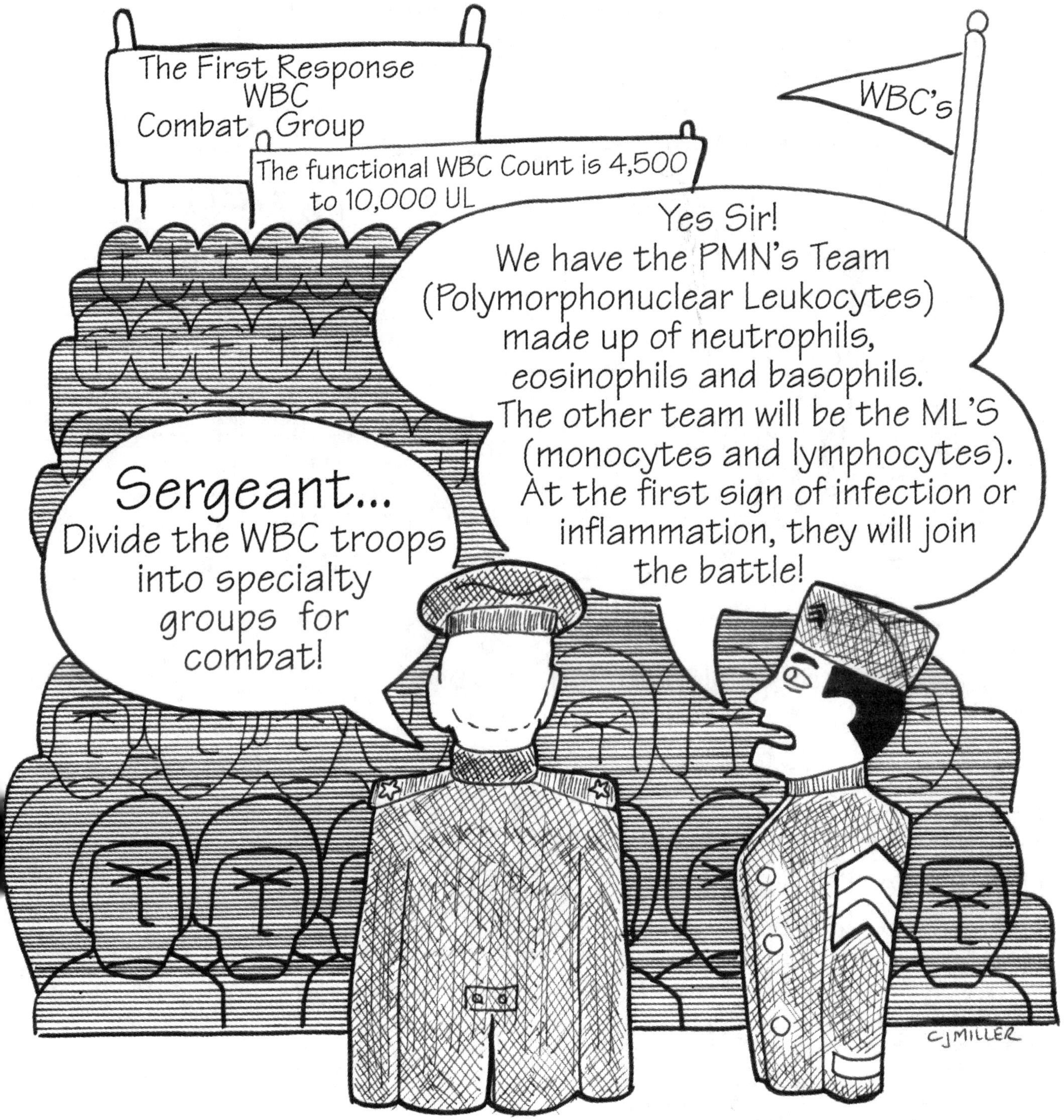
The First Response WBC Combat Group
WBC's
The functional WBC Count is 4,500 to 10,000 UL
Sergeant... Divide the WBC troops into specialty groups for combat!
Yes Sir! We have the PMN's Team (Polymorphonuclear Leukocytes) made up of neutrophils, eosinophils and basophils. The other team will be the ML'S (monocytes and lymphocytes). At the first sign of infection or inflammation, they will join the battle!
CJMILLER

Bone Densitometry

Bone Mineral Density

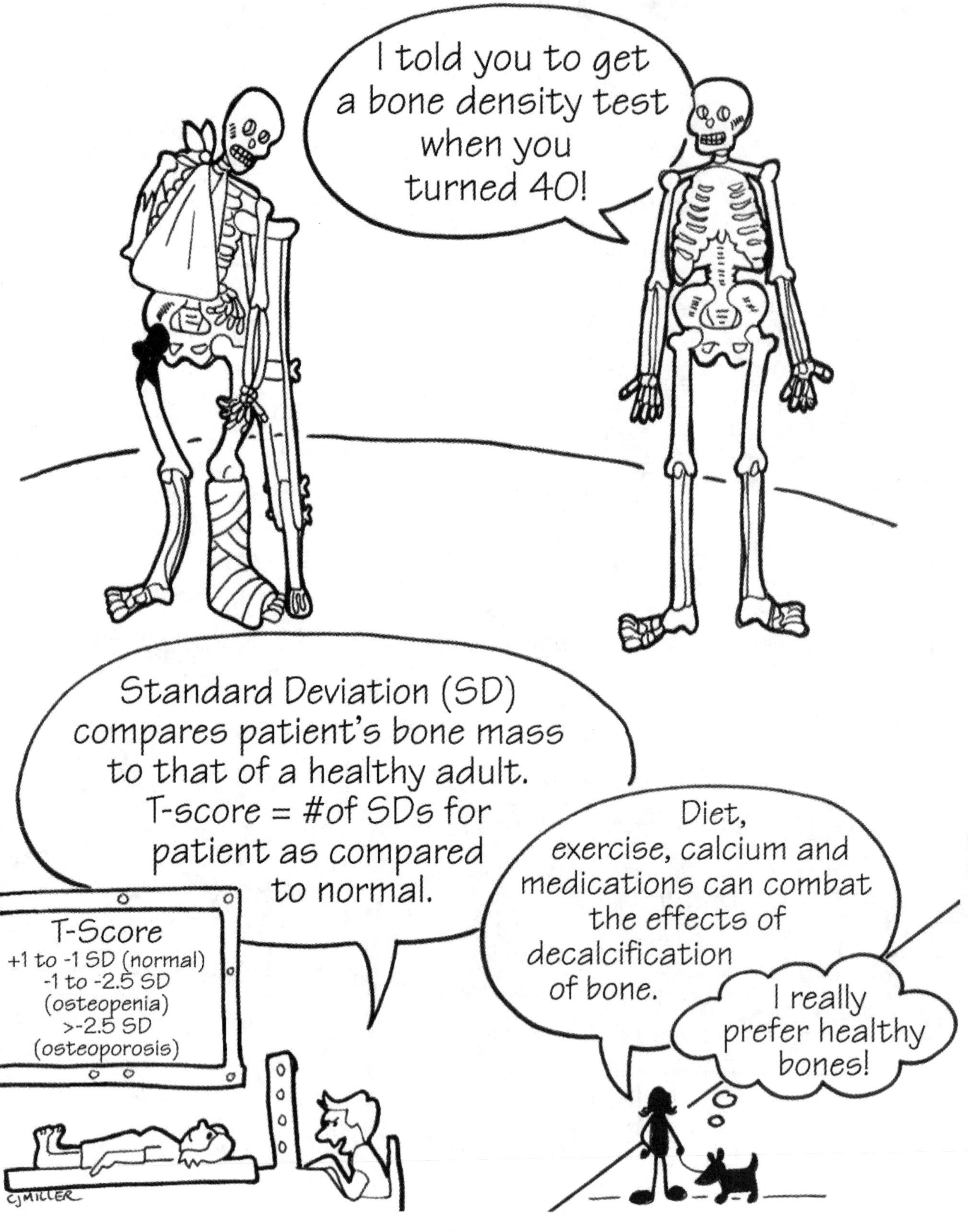

I told you to get a bone density test when you turned 40!
Standard Deviation (SD) compares patient's bone mass to that of a healthy adult. T-score = #of SDs for patient as compared to normal.
T-Score
+1 to -1 SD (normal)
-1 to -2.5 SD (osteopenia)
>-2.5 SD (osteoporosis)
Diet, exercise, calcium and medications can combat the effects of decalcification of bone.
I really prefer healthy bones!
CJMILLER

Bronchoscopy

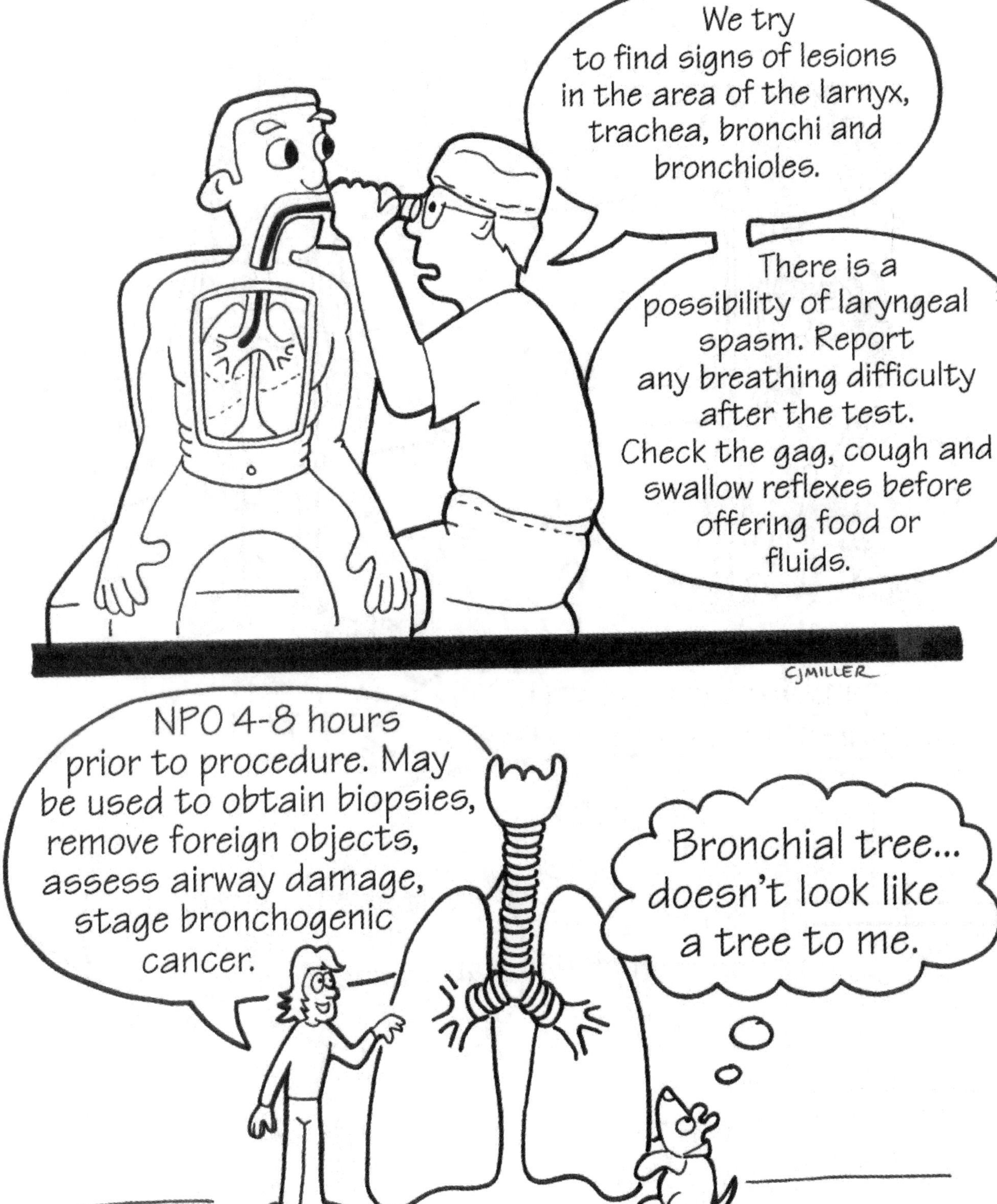
We try to find signs of lesions in the area of the larnyx, trachea, bronchi and bronchioles.
There is a possibility of laryngeal spasm. Report any breathing difficulty after the test. Check the gag, cough and swallow reflexes before offering food or fluids.
CJMILLER
NPO 4-8 hours prior to procedure. May be used to obtain biopsies, remove foreign objects, assess airway damage, stage bronchogenic cancer.
Bronchial tree... doesn't look like a tree to me.

Chorionic Villus Sampling (CVS)

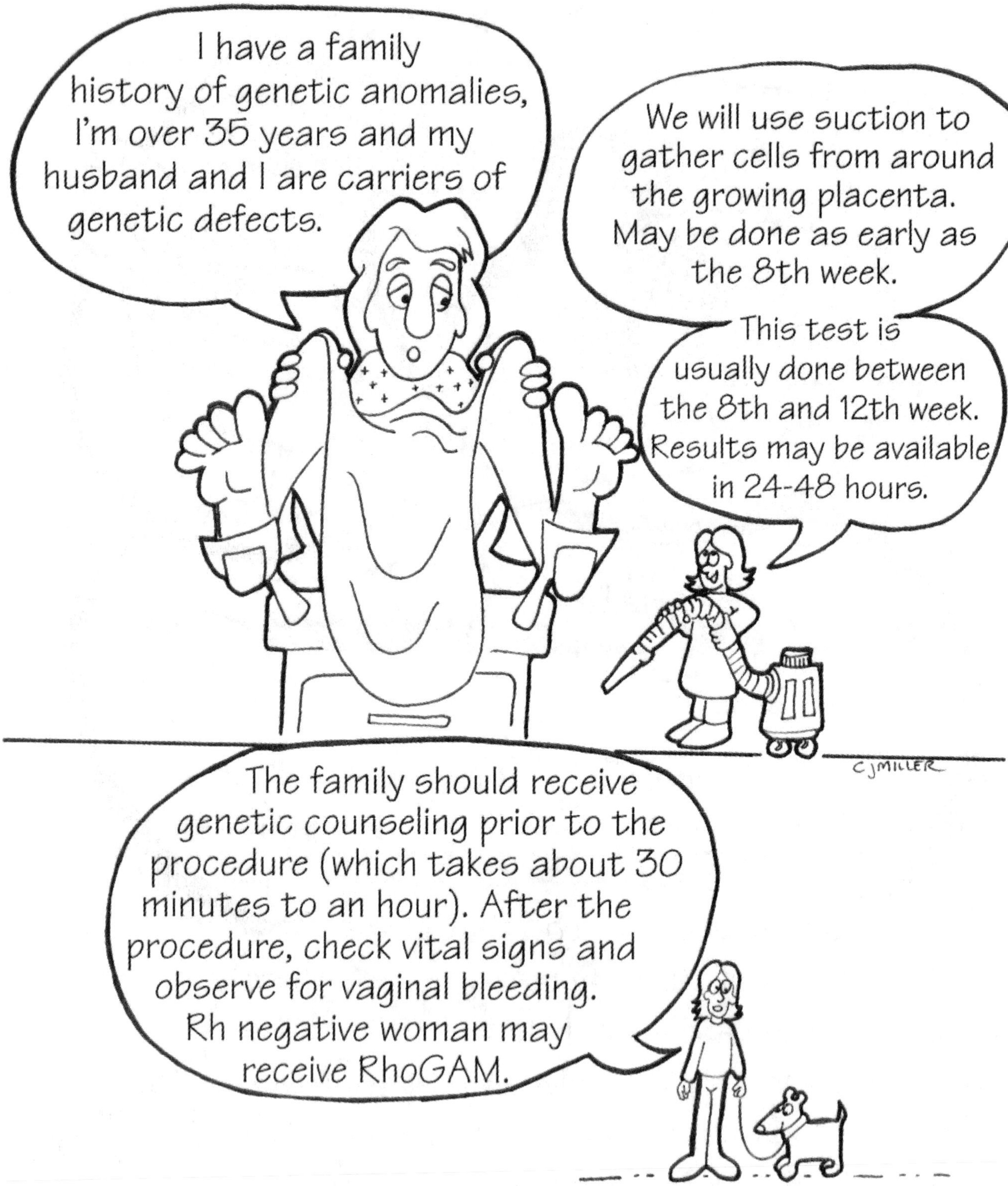

I have a family history of genetic anomalies, I'm over 35 years and my husband and I are carriers of genetic defects.
We will use suction to gather cells from around the growing placenta. May be done as early as the 8th week.
This test is usually done between the 8th and 12th week. Results may be available in 24-48 hours.
The family should receive genetic counseling prior to the procedure (which takes about 30 minutes to an hour). After the procedure, check vital signs and observe for vaginal bleeding. Rh negative woman may receive RhoGAM.
CJMILLER

Occult Blood

"Master Guaiac's Occult Blood"

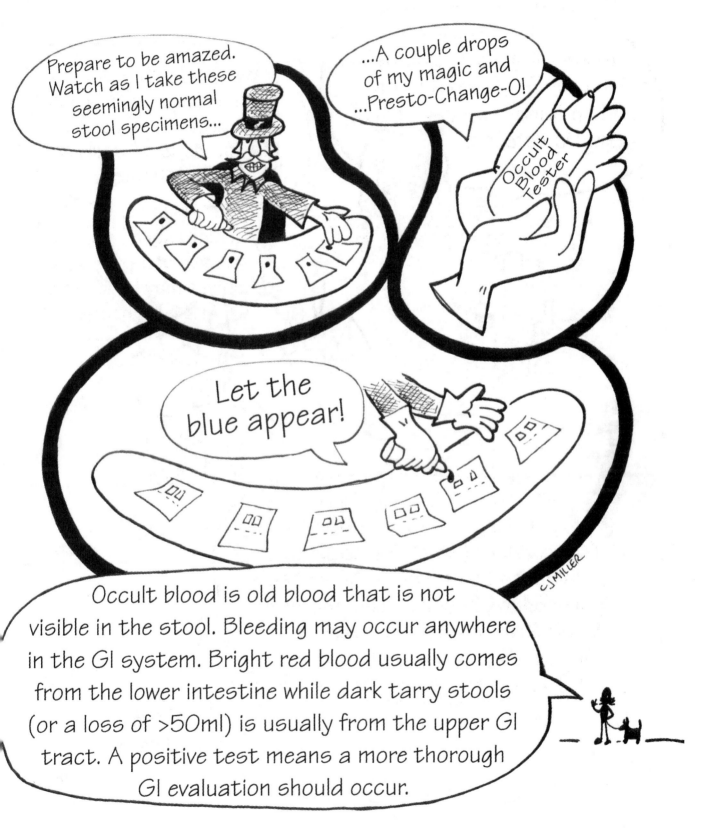

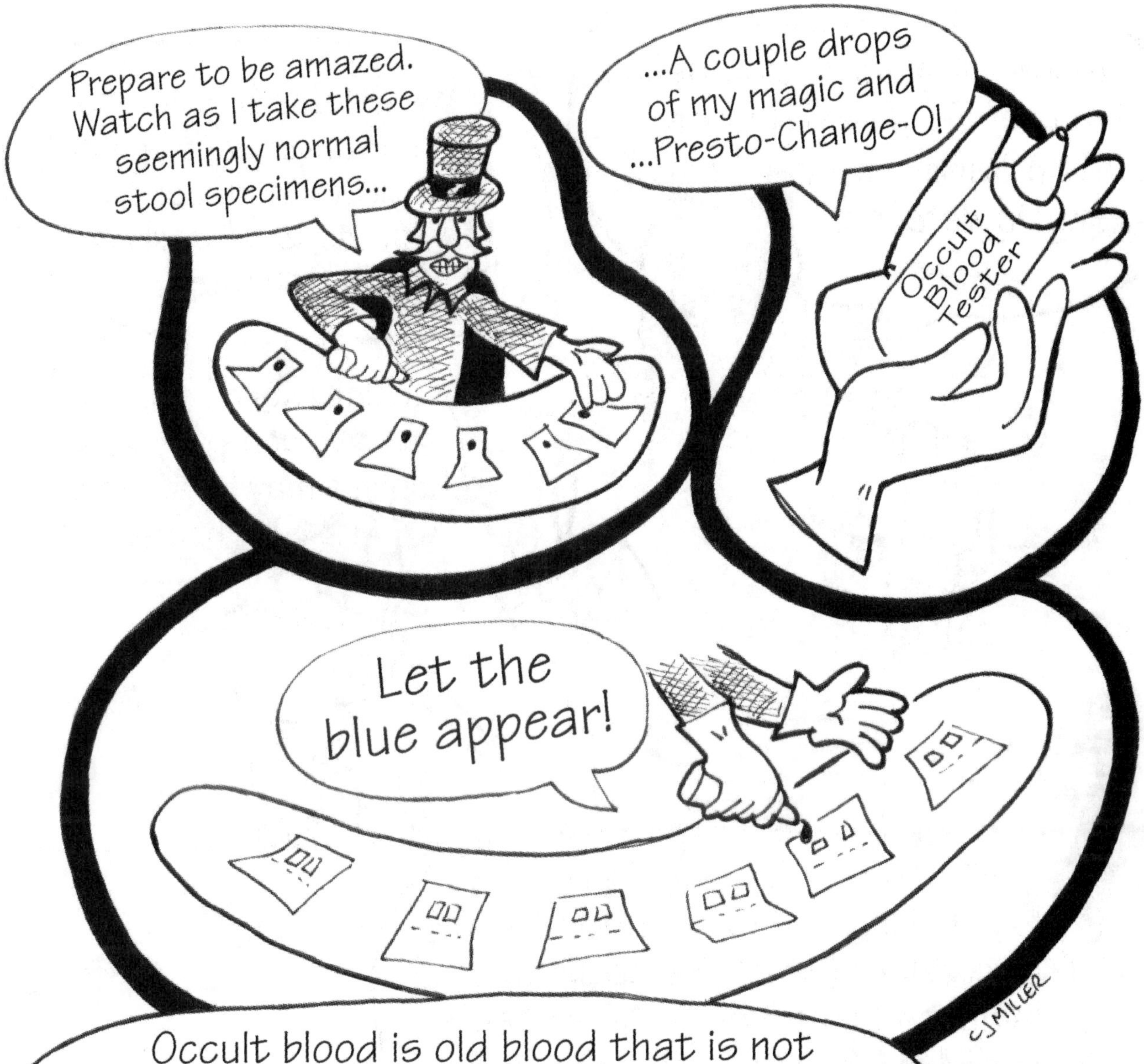
Prepare to be amazed. Watch as I take these seemingly normal stool specimens...
...A couple drops of my magic and ...Presto-Change-O!
Occult Blood Tester
Let the blue appear!
CJ MILLER

Occult blood is old blood that is not visible in the stool. Bleeding may occur anywhere in the GI system. Bright red blood usually comes from the lower intestine while dark tarry stools (or a loss of >50ml) is usually from the upper GI tract. A positive test means a more thorough GI evaluation should occur.

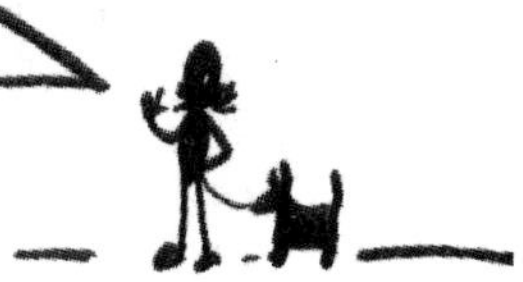

Spinal Fluid Analysis

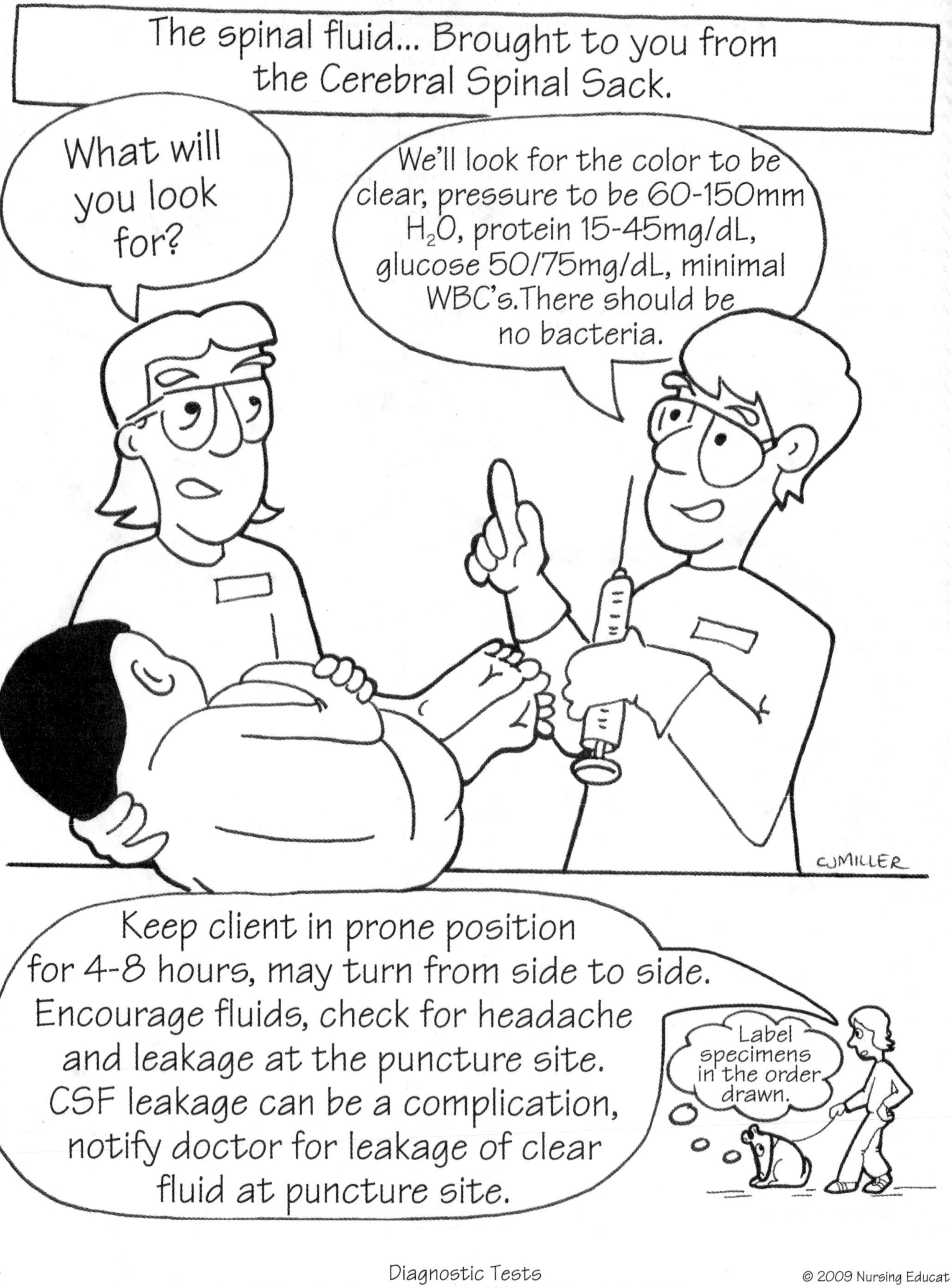

The spinal fluid... Brought to you from the Cerebral Spinal Sack.
What will you look for?
We'll look for the color to be clear, pressure to be 60-150mm H_2O, protein 15-45mg/dL, glucose 50/75mg/dL, minimal WBC's.There should be no bacteria.
CJMILLER
Keep client in prone position for 4-8 hours, may turn from side to side. Encourage fluids, check for headache and leakage at the puncture site. CSF leakage can be a complication, notify doctor for leakage of clear fluid at puncture site.
Label specimens in the order drawn.